Great Legs!

Great Legs!

Every Girl's Guide to Healthy, Sexy, Strong Legs

Jane Merrill

Andrews McMeel
Publishing

Kansas City

Great Legs!

05 06 07 08 09 MLT 10 9 8 7 6 5 4 3 2 1

ISBN-13: 978-0-7407-5486-9
ISBN-10: 0-7404-5486-6

Library of Congress Control Number: 2005047520

www.andrewsmcmeel.com

Book design by Diane Marsh

ATTENTION: SCHOOLS AND BUSINESSES

Andrews McMeel books are available at quantity discounts with bulk purchase for educational, business, or sales promotional use. For information, please write to: Special Sales Department, Andrews McMeel Publishing, 4520 Main Street, Kansas City, Missouri 64111.

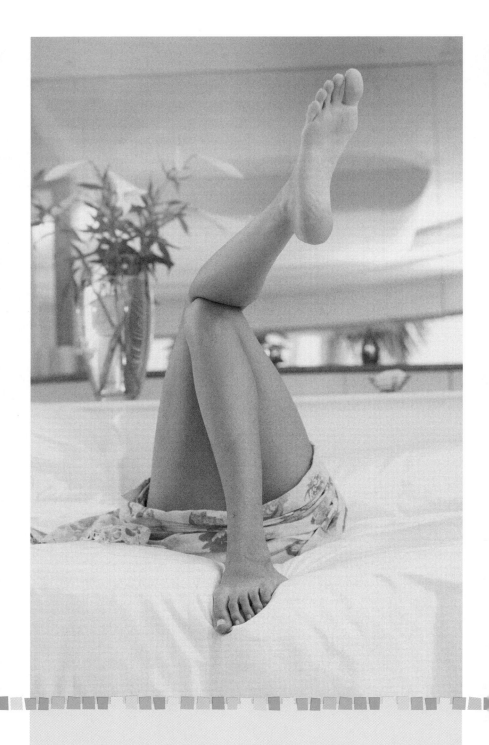

Contents

PART II *Feet*

Acknowledgments

THE SUBJECT OF beautiful legs is encyclopedic and includes much information that is brand-new. I had the generous help of medical specialists at the forefront of their fields. My gratitude goes to Dr. Mark Iafrati, vascular surgeon of Tufts–New England Medical Center; Dr. Joseph Pober, plastic surgeon; Dr. Andrew H. Rice, foot surgeon; Dr. Ron M. Shelton, of the New York Aesthetic Center; Dr. Mary Bove, doctor of naturopathic medicine in Brattleboro, Vermont; Dr. Celeste Romig, esteemed dermatologist in Darien, Connecticut; my friend Dr. Robert J. Terdiman, cardiologist; Dr. Kevin Plancher, orthopedic knee surgeon; Dr. Lionel Bissoon, president of the American Board of Mesotherapy; and Dr. Mark Ostreicher of Westport, Connecticut.

Sometimes people shared with me with such enthusiasm and alacrity that I went back to them to brainstorm as well as to verify. Fred Hahn, owner of Serious Strength in New York City; Ion Grumeza, trainer of gymnasts and boxers, author of a biography of the Olympic gold medalist Nadia Comaneci, and a certified fitness specialist at the YMCA of Westport, Connecticut; Melissa Hamilton of the Hands On Massage Therapy Center in Greenwich, Connecticut; Kymberlee Harris of Wolford Lingerie; Roberta Boyle of Green Valley Aromatherapy Ltd.; and Sue Setari, proprietor of Azena Salon and Douglas Parfumerie Cosmetics in Westport, Connecticut Aromatherapy were invaluable sources because they love what they do.

Early on, a lot of my bright questions came up with no answers. That's when I sought the help of several fine minds: Chris Filstrup, dean of the State University of New York at Stony Brook; Sherry Goodman, head of education at the University of California at Berkeley; Usha Bhasker at the New York Public Library; and Emma N. Filstrup, beginning her legal career in Washington, D.C.

Thanks to Jean Lucas, the best editor imaginable; Andrea Hurst, my literary agent, for helping conceptualize this book; Gary Stromberg for the benefit of his blazing imagination and ideas, extended with loving-kindness; Escence McCoy for her patient preparation of the manuscript; my brilliant editorial assistant at Colgate University, Matthew Fortin; and my friend Susan R. Romero, fashion reporter and attorney, who took time while completing her master's in journalism at Columbia to research like a dream.

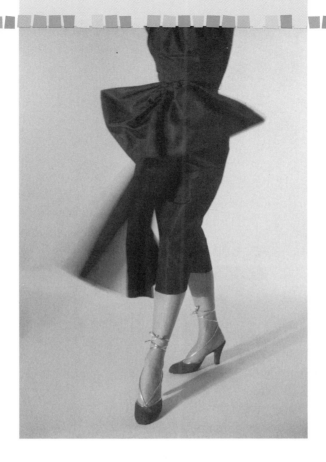

Introduction

LEGS HAVE ALWAYS been in style, even in the 1900s, when hemlines barely rose above the ankles. After skirts finally came up, in 1920, they rarely came down for long. Whatever the state of fashion, the sexy legs of movie stars, models, and sports figures are timeless.

The next decade was a fashion roller coaster. Hemlines went down in 1923, and then came up to the knees in 1925. By 1928 skirts were below the knee again. In the 1930s hemlines depressed with the economy, and Americans escaped to movies and shows. On screen, audiences got a glimpse of Jean Harlow, sans underwear, with her legs peeking out from slits in her white negligees. The ultimate leg candy, the Rockettes (originally the Roxyettes), came to Radio City Music Hall in 1932. This entire seventy-five-year-old show at Radio City Music Hall is built around women who form kick lines as a profession.

In the 1940s, World War II resulted in fabric rationing, and skirts became narrower and shorter, revealing more leg than ever. In the movies, Cyd Charisse and her long, lean legs danced across the floor with Fred Astaire, and Betty Grable, whose legs were insured for $1,250,000, posed for pinup shots in a bathing suit and high heels. "There are two reasons why I'm in show business, and I'm standing on both of them" is Grable's famous line. Legs were in, and stocking ads were bold, featuring pictures of women's legs in thigh-high stockings and garters. As if this was not enough, the bikini swimsuit was invented in 1946. By the late 1940s, the designer Christian Dior dashed the leg craze with his "New Look," featuring full calf-length skirts. Women protested Dior's collection with picket signs reading, "Keep 'Em Short" and "Protect the American Leg."

Dior's style reigned in the 1950s, when fabric rationing ended; films offered a reprieve from the disappearing leg, highlighted by Marilyn Monroe in her famous white halter dress standing over a street grating. By 1960, hemlines sky-rocketed when the London designer Mary Quant created the miniskirt and hot pants. Panty hose production more than tripled from 200 million in 1968 to 624 million in 1969, and models such as Twiggy and Veruschka helped to fuel the miniskirt explosion.

In the 1970s the mini and maxi skirts were both in vogue, yet legs stood their ground. Hemlines settled down in the 1980s, and pantsuits were in, but women's legs were still seen. *Dallas* and *Dynasty* dominated television, and the leading ladies—Linda Gray, Victoria Principal, Linda Evans, and Joan Collins—had classic great gams. Footwear was a crucial leg accessory in the 1990s, as skirts became slimmer and clothes had a more minimalist look. Manolo Blahnik and Jimmy Choo became footwear celebrities who made every leg look better in their pointed-toe, stiletto heels.

Today's skirts vary in length, and miniskirts and hot pants are back. The actresses Nicole Kidman and Cameron Diaz personify the millennium leg—long, taut, and fit. Women are buff, and the war on cellulite is raging. Hemlines show no sign of dropping—the American leg is protected.

A beauty revolution has begun. This revolution is responsible for the unprecedented availability of the leg makeover. European aristocrats' and Hollywood stars' painstaking treatments and their secret ingredients are out of the spa closet. Exercise gurus have body-part-specific workouts. Even inborn flaws, or unsightly leg features that are lifestyle-specific, can be altered. For example, calves can be made shapelier, fat pads on knees can be removed, and scars and discolorations of the leg can be erased. Yet how relatively unknown these awesome treatments are! Women's magazines cover everything from pedicure products and depilatories to seasonal exercises to slim down thighs. But you'd never even sense from their articles or advertisements how much leg health and beauty have advanced beyond nail polish and pumice stones. All the information you need for your own leg makeover is included in *Great Legs!*

The treatments explained in this book go from the traditional and homespun to the "spa-torial" of the highest technology. The array of marvelous products available to make legs and feet silky smooth will amaze you. Improved laser and X-ray diagnostics, curative injections, and a range of dermatological and vascular treatments are more amazing still. There's no question that you can have stronger and prettier legs than you ever thought possible. Begin by taking a long, steady look to evaluate your legs for strength and beauty, and to determine where you need to get active to grow more beautiful.

It used to be quipped that, of a woman's attractions, legs were the "last to go." Today we have wondrous medical treatments so our legs can be pretty when we're old, and even stronger. Moreover, we can do simple exercises on a gym ball, on a mat, or with straight-backed chairs that help maintain and enhance our legs' youthful shapeliness and muscularity. Had our mothers only known. Legs don't ever have to go!

Unfortunately, we damage our legs without meaning to or even being aware we do it. We stand far too long "at attention" at our jobs. We don the wrong shoes until our calves bow and our feet bleed and cramp like those of the Wicked Witch of the West. We have pregnancies without considering the effect of an extra twenty-five to forty pounds on our legs and feet. We undertrain and overdo in sports, pushing our bodies and punishing our legs. Some of us suffer from protruding and "spider" veins, red dots, moles, and discoloration; some complain, some don't. Either way, we wish these conditions didn't mar our looks.

So don't put up with callused feet and red, roughened ankles, or give up on your slender thighs that have turned to jelly. Resolve these problems and have *flawless legs*. The proven treatments are here; you only have to know what you're doing. Here you'll learn about the relation between nutrition and circulation, creams and baths, commercial products and herbal remedies, and high-tech medical procedures. If you want a spa pedicure, you can learn how to get one without stepping out of your house. If you take care of yourself, you want to be better informed. Here you'll find all the wisdom and information required, at the lowest cost and for the greatest legs. This book will cover legs, knees, and

"A girls' face may be her fortune, but it's her legs that draw the interest." The most celebrated legs in history include the following:

- Josephine Baker (seen very naked)
- Betty Grable (seen in sweetheart poses)
- Lauren Bacall (looking très chic)
- Marilyn Monroe (in ultrasexy poses)
- Ann Miller (in the motion of dance)
- Jane Russell (colorfully costumed)
- Katharine Hepburn (seen through flowing gowns)
- Tina Turner (too remarkable a singer to have such fantastic legs)
- Beyoncé Knowles (ditto)
- Cindy Crawford (glamorously long)
- Sophia Loren (so ladylike)
- Audrey Hepburn (twiggy but good tone)
- Charlize Theron (the perfect model's)
- Vanessa Williams (ideal strength)
- Patti LaBelle
- Steffi Graf
- Daryl Hannah

These are just a few of the most celebrated legs of all time. If you follow my simple instructions, you could have great legs, too!

feet. From heavy-duty vascular-dermatological procedures to day-to-day prevention, from exercises that can be done at your desk or while driving to alternative therapies, from Mother Nature's secrets to supplements and nutritional information, all are included here. So put up your legs, and think pretty!

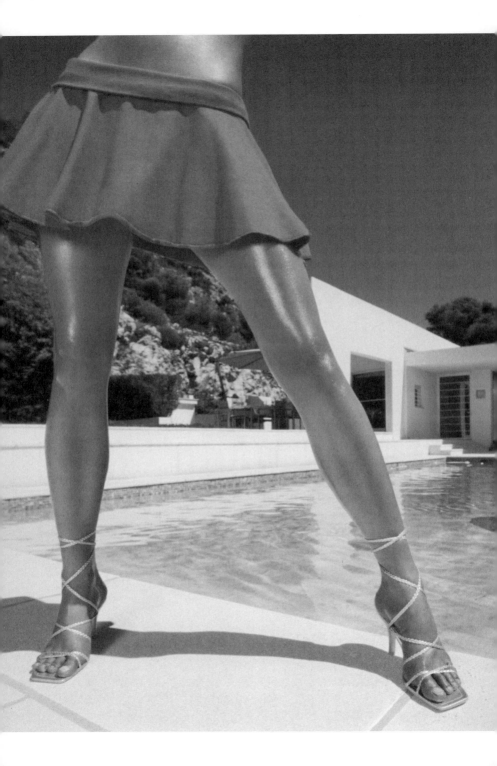

PART I

Legs

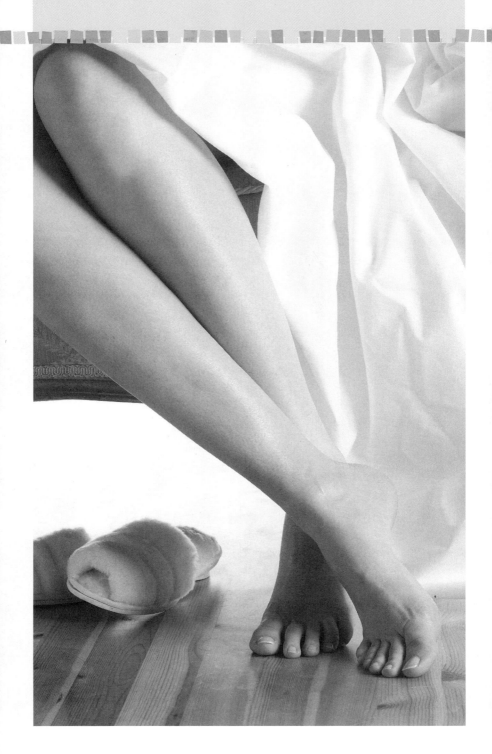

$\mathcal{L}eg\ \mathcal{C}are$

HOME SPA TREATMENTS

If your face is like a delicate flower, your legs are your trees. Trees need water, soil, and sun just like flowers, but they don't need care nearly so often. If you do a home spa treatment once a week, it's plenty. How about Friday when you get home from work, with a friend instead of meeting for coffee on Saturday, or while you read the Sunday newspaper? Home and professional spa treatments are not either-or. Take advantage of a good day spa, try out the touted one on vacation, but if your time or money is limited, buy some basic tools and products, and enjoy a spa treatment in your own home. Okay, so you can't just lie back and close your eyes the whole time, but need I point out that your feet and legs will not feel shortchanged!

I confess, I'm an ex–bath product junkie. In my time I've filled a shopping cart with bubble bath, beads, shower gels, and sprays. Was it growing up on a stern regimen of soap and water that made me do it? Some women like to experiment with makeup, some of us go for what smells and feels good. In stores we study bottles like cooks before a grocery shelf of salsas.

Here are some companies with the most ravishing lines for legs and unique, high-quality products you might want to try: Kneipp has been around for over one hundred years and is a trusted name throughout Europe. It is a German-based bath and body company that uses herbs and plants to achieve a sense of overall wellness. Kneipp is to bath products what Guerlain and Chanel are to perfumes. Now my baths are tinted jewel-like colors, and unlike all the candles that claim to engender peace or arousal, Kneipp products actually do promote the moods promised. You find yourself treasuring a Kneipp bath or shower product, and you can use it sparingly, because the formula is pure and concentrated. As the thermal bath salts exfoliate, you may feel them increase your skin's elasticity. Wow, just like the package says! Everything comes in six or seven herbal scents.

The line that features the *Arnica montana* flower is pure indulgence. Arnica is used in all the Kneipp leg products for its soothing and cooling properties. This bright yellow daisy-like flower blooms around July and is indigenous to Europe, southern Russia, and central Asia. *Arnica montana* flower has been known for centuries for its antiseptic and painkilling properties. Try their Arnica Leg Cream after strenuous exercise or a long day on your feet. Massage your feet and ankles to midthigh using upward movements. Because of the astringent arnica, the cream and other products are way above the ordinary. Both the cream and the gel help with circulation and are said to reduce puffiness.

The Kneipp Herbal Bath comes in nine scents that satisfy different minds and bodies. For instance, rosemary is known to be invigorating and wakes up the system. Romans viewed the rosemary wreath as a symbol of energy. Spruce lifts the senses, while melissa is relaxing and good for a sound sleep.

Ever since Erica Jong wrote her volume of fruit and vegetable sexy poetry, we've been besieged with natural cosmetics we can make in our own kitchens. Not mine, though, where you may find a cucumber when your eyes are sore but not an avocado when your legs are dry. And I'm not baking pine nuts to exfoliate, since I consider my best trick staying out of the kitchen as much as I do yet raising four healthy children.

I sew and tend a garden, but I don't quarter pineapples to smoosh over my skin in the shower. (Think of the plumbing repairs.) My cosmetics cabinet is full of products in pretty jars, tubes, and bottles. The only reason I put cucumber on my eyelids or use an egg and oatmeal face mask is because I'm out of my favorite product.

The leg cosmetics routine can be done either with store-bought products or with ingredients you have on hand. Read the label because the contents vary radically from product to product. For instance:

- Bath additives laced with iodine-rich algae and seaweed condition the skin while balancing energy levels, slimming and toning the body, and relieving joint pain.

- Pure sea salts harvested from the mineral-laden Dead Sea offer high concentrations of sodium, magnesium, potassium, calcium, and phosphorus—essential nutrients for a well-functioning body. "The chemical composition of seaweed and seawater is similar to that of blood plasma and when used in the bath, soothes and heals the skin," notes Julie Sheikman, an aesthetician with Zia Natural Skincare in San Francisco. A cheap bath that is nice to the skin is a simple mix of half a box of baking soda and a cup of sea salt. Kosher salt is better for a paste with olive oil. Start with 2 tablespoons of the kosher salt, and add 1 tablespoon or a little more of the olive oil. (The extravirgin type is said to be a deoxidizing agent.)

- Evening primrose oil is cultivated from the vivid yellow evening primrose flower and aids in beautifying the skin through its anti-inflammatory properties. It is powerfully nurturing and moisturizing.

- Calendula, more commonly known as marigold, will heal, sooth, and relieve. Calendula's primary active compounds include anti-inflammatory agents as well as astringent and antiseptic properties. It is recommended as a primary ingredient in lotions to prevent shaving burn.

HOME SPA ROUTINE

Whether you have a huge claw-foot tub or one with an overhead sprayer, it's important that your bathroom is equipped to provide a private spa experience. To take advantage of this rite of health, include the following routine as often as you can during the week.

1. CLEANSE AND TONE. Start off by dipping in the tub, to relax your joints and muscles, and to alleviate the dryness of your skin. (You may skip this total immersion if you're doing a home spa treatment with a girlfriend. In that case, wash your legs with a European-style hand shower or just a very drippy washcloth from a basin of water and something nice like a dissolved bath bead.) Dissolve your bath beads or bath oil as directed on the package. Cheap is fine. I often use Vaseline, Walgreens, or Spa Magik's bath beads, which are 100 percent Dead Sea salts. At a better pharmacy or directly from the supplier you can find the marvelous Kneipp jewel-hued and intense bath oils, from Juniper to Chamomile. You'll feel better already after this textured dip. Just don't dunk in your head, as the treated water will coat your hair, too. Pat your legs dry; you'll get back to them later. You're going to break now for your feet!

2. EXFOLIATE. Gentle exfoliation before soaking will enhance the absorption of bath additives, be they detoxifying or hydrating. Dr. Adrienne Denese, a Manhattan antiaging medicine specialist, states that "dry brushing stimulates the lymphatic system." Scrub-a-dub, buff your feet with a foot scrub. The best foot scrubs are loaded with pumice, seaweed extract, apricot kernel oils, and ground walnut shells. The idea is to exfoliate and soothe. Dr. Denese states that you should start at the toes and work up the legs, using short, stimulating strokes with a natural-fiber brush. This step is what works the real magic, and is what you pay big bucks for at the spa.

Great Legs!

Exfoliants have a trio of ingredients: sea salts, oils, and moisturizers. They take years off the condition of your feet! Dr. Denese cautions that exfoliating products should never be used after a bath. "After soaking, the skin becomes soft, and it's possible to exfoliate too deeply," she says.

3. SOAK. Put your feet in a basin with a footbath like Get Fresh's Totally Soaked Soy Foot Bath. Don't be a skeptic; this is not just a feel-good step. A good footbath has ingredients specifically designed to dissolve dead skin cells and soften calluses as well as leave a protective sheen on your feet. I use Eskandar Milky Bath Soaks, which turn water milky white and generate a mild froth to cleanse the skin. Five minutes will do the trick.

4. APPLY A MASK. This step should be done every week—or as often as you feel your feet going back to their old frazzled, grizzly selves and your legs bearing the weight of the world. A foot mask nourishes and repairs your skin's layers. You leave it on for about five minutes. Stuff like fruit acids, algae extracts, and skin-softening oils give an intensive foot treatment that will make such a difference you will happily add it to your regimen. During these five minutes you will also do something very important: perform some massage tricks that are therapeutic and that your legs are going to love.

5. MASSAGE. Kneading your feet gently is going to expel the toxins that run through your body's lymphatic system. The other way to detox is with aerobics or yoga, which are covered in the Exercises section. You're working superficial tissues, so don't think vigorous, think lazy. Slow rubbing, squeezing movements that pull the toxins from your body are also part of the pinpointed weight-loss regimen to get rid of fat on your calves, knees, or thighs. To banish every final tiredness and ache from even the weariest legs and feet, try

hitting three points with ten seconds each of pressure: behind the knees, halfway down the calves, and at the base of the ankles. Once you've finished with the massage, rinse and dry your legs.

6. BUTTER UP. Choose a product with shea butter, or a rich, buttery moisturizing cream. Apply it thickly to the front and back of your legs. Put on a pair of booties (from a yoga supply store) or wrap your feet in plastic wrap and slip on your slippers. Leave the butter on until it's absorbed. The yoga booties, also called foot mittens, have a layer of herbs sewn in, so eventually you will want to get a pair. If you like the idea, get the electric booties. Women do a similar thing to pamper their hands with latex gloves, but I think doing that feels too Gloria Swanson. You certainly can slough, buff, and moisturize your hands for double benefit of the spa session, though.

If you are continuing with your day after this process, you might want to wait ten minutes and then with a washcloth remove the body butter and put on something light and rapidly absorbed, like Roger & Gallet's Green Tea Body Lotion.

The Caffeine Treatment is another highly effective kitchen-made regimen that I enjoy. For this you use the same hand massage but do it in the shower after you apply a paste of Dunkin' Donuts coffee, olive oil, and (optional) old-fashioned oatmeal. Proportions are inconsequential, so long as you end up with a sticky mess. Rub it on your thighs and legs. If you want to use a self-tanner, apply it after this wake-up call to your skin and it will take better. As I said before, my attitude toward all kitchen beauty products is very skeptical. However, several of my friends have had amazing results with the Caffeine Treatment. Try it three times a week and see.

Regardless of the products you use, please see that your home spa is an intimate one, one you don't share with anybody else. Do we always have to look outside ourselves for fulfillment? Imagine giving *yourself* the gift that's fulfilling and luxurious. The amazing fact of this experience is that you are caring for your outside as well as your inside. And remember that, no matter how decadent you make it, it's still positively beneficial for you.

LOTION TRANSITION

Are you as perplexed as I was about why we apply face creams religiously and totally neglect our legs? Well, I talked to many women, and we figured out what inhibits us from doing right by our legs in our beauty routines. The culprit is body lotions that come in pastel containers tied with ribbons and bearing flowery labels that you get in gift baskets or on sale at the pharmacy and that sit there unused.

We'll turn the body lotion containers into lamp bases or bud vases, because the lotions are almost certain to be gooey, greasy, and sticky, as well as having an overpowering chemical smell. You opened one once; remember how your good intentions dissolved when you put the gunk on? As few as one in one hundred lotions on the market have ingredients that will truly soften your skin and leave a silky smooth barrier to protect it from changes in temperature and humidity that cause dryness and roughness.

Read the labels and eliminate lotions with lanolin, which tends to suffocate. The best bath and body products contain natural formulas to exfoliate, stimulate, and create a protective barrier that will last throughout the day. Look for three types of ingredients: antioxidants and vitamin C, uncommon oils that decongest the skin, and "serious" creams to condition and moisturize. The more "designer" products will boast their plant, mineral, herb, and flower ingredients. You'll feel the difference when lotions with no artificial chemicals touch and penetrate your skin. In the Shopping Guide at the end of the book, you'll find recommendations for lotions that will make you want to use them daily, as you should. Some of my favorite lines are Roger & Gallet, Spa Magik, Eskandar, Caswell-Massey, and Get Fresh. There are often free samples available to those who shop online. I suggest choosing one of these lines that has it all for legs and feet so you can carry out a trial for yourself.

Factors like climate, whether you tan your legs, and how much natural oil your skin has will cause you to embrace one as just right. Do you wear perfume daily? If so, you also want to layer a moisturizer and bath products that complement the rosy, citrusy, or spicy base of your perfume.

LUXURY SPA TIPS

When buying a foaming bath, look for a cocoa or shea butter base. Most brands of bubble bath are drying; if you use bubble bath often, add a teaspoon of bath oil. Also be sure to look for concentrated forms of seawater, because of its vitamins and minerals and intense hydrating properties. Some products include Detoxifying Seaweed Bath, available at www.espaonline.com, and Repêchage Vita Cura Seaweed Bath, available at www.repechage.com.

A trick to exfoliate without toil is to get the fiber gloves from Parfums Mary Douglas. They come in bright colors and cost a few dollars. Take an exfoliating cream or soap, put the gloves on, rub the cream into the legs, and feel how invigorating it can be.

Salt glows can be used after you cleanse, separately or in a product that includes them. The sodium draws impurities and excess water from your body.

Do not use massage oil to moisturize your legs and feet. Therapeutic massage oil won't be absorbed. You want to moisturize with a softener-moisturizer designed for this purpose.

Loofahs are good! They feel good and stimulate the skin. Use your loofah to scrub everywhere and see your skin glow. Apply body gel or seaweed soap with the loofah. Use the loofah a few times; wring it out and dry it each time. Then throw it away.

If you find a product you like and don't see it again or want to check out more products in the line, find it on amazon.com. Say you have a discontinued Estée Lauder cosmetic; search for it. Discontinued beauty salon products are available on the Internet. It's nice to see products displayed and have them personally endorsed by aestheticians who use them, and you can get very reasonable prices online.

Try Saks, Nordstrom, or Macy's for a foot and leg care kit. The small sizes give you a taste of new items. Take for

Great Legs!

instance the kit from Get Fresh. This is packed with ingredients like seaweed, shea butter, pumice, soy, and fruit acids, and it includes foot spray, scrub, mask, footbath, and a wonderful Rescue Me Foot Repair Cream.

To know if a lymphatic massage is the real McCoy, see what training is purported and whether it is a series (which it should be to work), and check out the referrals. After you've had a lymphatic massage, cut down a bit on salt and fatty foods and drink enough water. Do this for several days and it will turn out to be much more beneficial.

MILK BATHS

"They say that milk improves the skin, but drink it, dear, don't rub it in!" This old rhyme used to stop girls from going to the icebox for a treat for their skin. The gentle AHA (alpha hydroxy acid) found in milk is good for the skin; it penetrates and hydrates. It also helps remove the old top layer and leaves the bloom of fresh skin. It promotes the elasticity of the upper layer of skin and makes it softer. For a more potent formula, you can get a body or leg product with 4 or more percent of an AHA (glycol is the strongest, used on wrinkles) or one advertised as having a lot of "fruit acids."

The lactic acid in milk has a softening effect. Is it the mystique that makes you glow after a milk bath? I feel like a duchess. Do not rinse off, nothing will curdle! Mix a cup of instant powdered milk into the bathwater as you fill the tub, then add 4 drops of peppermint or almond oil.

RECIPE FOR A HOME MILK BATH

1 cup powdered milk
1 cup ground oatmeal (use a blender or food processor)
1 cup baking soda
1 cup Epsom salts
15–20 drops lavender essential oil
      (for a calming, stress-relieving bath)
Or 10 drops rose, jasmine, or neroli essential oil
      (for a sensual bath; these oils are known aphrodisiacs)

Blend together really well in a glass or stainless steel bowl (plastic will take on the scent of the oils), and store in an airtight glass jar. Use 12 ounces per bath.

You can also purchase your milk bath already formulated. It is the milk that will make your skin creamy smooth, so be sure the milk is more than just in the name! Caswell-

Massey's Old Fashioned Milk Bath has a fresh, evocative hyacinth fragrance. See what's in it: extracts of ivy, arnica, and cucumber; aloe; and milk proteins and whole milk. The most popular body lotion from Caswell-Massey, Almond & Aloe, has sweet almond oil (to moisturize), aloe vera gel (for healing), and extracts of chamomile (to soften), hyssop and rosemary (to relax), and calendula (to soothe).

Lactic acid in milk baths and glycolic acid in sugarcane, or the kelp my aunt used to throw in the bath as well as in our soup, can keep skin soft and smooth. However, Dr. Mark Ostreicher, foot surgeon and professor at Yale Medical School, notes that natural and prescription-strength products are often the best. One or 2 percent of people will experience irritation from a substance; high potency is what can be so good for us but can also be allergenic. Commercial products, whether pricey or cheap, have low levels of the beneficial ingredient so they don't cause irritation. If you have very sensitive skin, instead of absorbing the goodies in the bathwater, take Dr. Ostreicher's advice. Get out and dry, and while your skin is still moist, use a prescription product that will give your skin a treat without being absorbed. He recommends products with alphalipoic or hyaluronic acid or coenzyme Q_{10}.

You can make a brisk shower or relaxing bath a beauty regimen for your legs. Sometimes we are in the mood for efficiency, sometimes we like to sink into luxury. Either way you can get creative with products and set the scene with whimsy or romance, or just get a kit from Get Fresh, Bliss, or Caswell-Massey that has all the goods for feet and legs. The thing to remember is this kind of beauty treatment works over time—it's not like changing your hair color or getting a manicure presto. You have to assemble the ingredients as if you were whipping up dessert, and go through your regimen consistently at least twice a week, month after month, to maintain great gams.

SCRUB!

Legs need the dry skin to be scrubbed off more than other parts of your body. Try massaging a guy's legs and feet and you'll feel as if you are using a very soft eraser. The cells virtually peel off. Imagine how important this step of your bathing routine is to keep your feminine skin soft and supple.

Each day your body sheds around 500 million dead cells from the upper epidermis. Some need a push from you to slough off. That's where body scrubs and body polishes, salt- or sugar-based scrubs, and bath paraphernalia such as brushes and loofahs come in. Exfoliation is an often-neglected step after cleansing your skin. Why is exfoliation a necessary self-care routine? If you let it go, especially if you keep lathing on moisturizers, your skin will start to appear dull and flaky.

Scrubbing or applying an exfoliating product should be done every day or at least several times a week in the summer, a little less often in the winter. Besides rejuvenating the skin on your legs and feet, it increases the circulation and loosens ingrown hair follicles before they cause trouble.

The mechanical way is to scrub with a loofah or a rough washcloth. Put a gel on your legs first. The spa-type alternative is to use a product intended for exfoliating. There are sugar, nut, and salt scrubs, but some products combine these elements. With the "scrub" range of products, you don't have to apply a lot of pressure or friction, just leave on the appointed minute or two and rinse off with your hands. These products are good for traveling even if you use a loofah at home.

The most important thing to remember is that no creams or potions can penetrate your skin unless, several times a week, you scrub! You can do it with sea salt or brown sugar exfoliators, or simply scrub. But remember, scrubbing is the sine qua non of leg beauty.

MOISTURIZING

We subject our legs to rapid changes in temperature and humidity, damaging sun rays, chafing from garments, and baths in hard water. Keeping your legs moisturized is not just a matter of keeping them soft. You want the moisturizer to penetrate. We put on heavy-duty moisturizer in the winter, when the heating system dries out legs, then forget about them. Do what's right to hydrate your poor wintry legs and feet year-round by using lotions and oils. Lotions are for nighttime, after a bath, after shaving, and after exposure to the sun. They are to be used lavishly. The texture of the lotion says a lot about how it will work on legs. It should be slick, not gummy. It should glide. It should be rich but not oily or separated. The better lotions usually have a subtle, distinctive fragrance that catches your imagination.

And here's a *jar* of oil,
just like in the Bible.
Lie in my arms,
I'll make your *flesh* glisten.

—Leonard Cohen, "I Have Two Bars of Soap"

THE BARE ESSENTIALS

As for essential oils and the legs, there are many beneficial possibilities. One of the first things to think about is circulation, especially if you are sitting at a desk or standing in one spot for the majority of the day.

Salt scrubs are a great way to rev up the circulation, especially combined with peppermint, black pepper, ginger, or rosemary oils for an extra boost. Blend 2 cups of base oil (like sweet almond or jojoba) and 3 cups of salt or sugar. Add a total of 20 drops of the abovementioned oils, and mix well. This blend should be applied to damp legs and rubbed from ankle to thigh (always toward the heart, to help the circulation). Rub for just *one* minute on each leg, then shower off. Your legs will feel smooth, refreshed, and revitalized!

One thing you want to internalize is that essential oils are not oily; they are usually steam-distilled from leaves, flowers, roots, wood, or peel and should not be used on the skin until they are blended into a carrier oil or base. This dilution will minimize the risk of a skin reaction. *Essential* just means that these oils are the "essence" or "lifeblood" of their plants. When you rub your hand over plants such as lavender or basil, the scent that lingers on your skin is the essential oil. Different plants offer different therapeutic benefits. Here is an overview of the different types: Lavender is relaxing (paradoxically, in large amounts it is a stimulant); orange, lemon, and grapefruit are uplifting; geranium is balancing; sandalwood is a sedative; rose and jasmine are known aphrodisiacs. You will feel these effects if you select products of quality, like Kneipp or Erbaviva.

With natural fragrances that you put in the bath or use as massage oil, it really is worth the trouble to purchase from mail-order suppliers or specialty stores to get the freshest, best distilled or extracted essential oils. With massage oils, the base oil to which the fragrance is added can be kept safely for up to six months. The best carrier oil, fine and not greasy, is

Great Legs!

almond oil. For greatest potency, the fragrances must be mixed in directly from the dropper right before you use them.

Aromatherapy is part science, part art, and you can find many books explaining it. Not everyone who wants beautiful legs has time to indulge is this subtle enhancement to a beauty regimen. So here is a summary of what I use the essences for and why. I have left out all the flowery sweet essences, on the assumption that more brisk scents should waft up from one's legs. Each of these can be mixed, so play chemist!

ESSENTIAL OILS DELECTABLE FOR YOUR LEGS (AND BODY)

ROSE GERANIUM Relaxing and calming, a little spicy. Add 8 drops to the bath just before you immerse.

EUCALYPTUS Refreshing and disinfecting, warms aching muscles. This is the only essence in my list that is exotic. The extract from the leaves and twigs of the gum tree comes from Australia and New Zealand.

LAVENDER Sprinkle fresh lavender sprigs in the bath. In small amounts it is relaxing. In large amounts it can be restorative and mood lifting.

JUNIPER Another strong essence, lovely for the bath and massage, with a special use as a rubdown to reduce cellulite.

PEPPERMINT Stimulating and antiseptic for a footbath. Use sparingly as it is more potent than many other essences. Put 1 drop of peppermint and 2 drops of lavender oil in the carrier oil as a massage oil that both men and women will like.

JASMINE More expensive than the other essences, because thousands of blossoms are required to furnish a teaspoon of it.

Jasmine is heady and not to be missed, but you can get it only from certain suppliers. When using it, consider going half and half with rose geranium for a spicy note. Both of these are known aphrodisiacs.

LEMON AND GRAPEFUIT Uplifting effect.

SANDALWOOD Sedative or calming effect.

The only way to make fragrance subtle is to layer. You wear the fragrance, it doesn't wear you. You bathe or shower, pat dry, and while the skin is moist, seal with a moisturizer, all in the same fragrance. In France, when a scent is obvious, it's called *les cuisses de ma tante* (my aunt's buttocks), overpowering.

HAIR REMOVAL OPTIONS

For now, many of us stay with the tried and true; however, the question is not *which method* of hair removal will give you satisfaction but how respectful you are to your skin!

RAZOR IT OFF This method is quick and not messy (unless you nick, which usually doesn't happen if you use a good razor with a clean, nonrusty blade). You can do it in the shower. Most women shave every other or every third day. If you have regrowth the next day and are zealous about no stubble, so much shaving will dry out your skin. Use an ointment for extra dry skin before you step into the shower. Then as soon as you get out, reapply it so it sinks in before you put on your clothes.

Creams with calendula are said to help with red bumps after shaving. Spas use tea tree oil *before* (and sometimes after) waxing to help disinfect and slightly numb the skin, but it can also help stop hair follicles from getting infected. Kiehl's sells several fantastic shaving lotions with ingredients including benzocaine, which is well known for its soothing and cooling properties, and azulene, which comes from the chamomile flower and is known for its cooling and healing properties.

WIPE IT OFF Depilatories now come in creams of pleasant fragrances and in sprays. If you used to sicken at the smell, try again; not only has the odor become more palatable but it doesn't waft around where it was used anymore. The directions usually specify 10 minutes maximum, so be sure to watch that clock. If the depilatory misses some hair, wait two days and use it again for half the time. Depilatories don't cause as many ingrown hairs as shaving because the regrowth tends to be fine wisps. All depilatories put the epidermis under stress. After you remove the product completely with wet paper towels or a cloth, rinse one more time and then take a bath with an extra dose of bath oil. The addition of a bath helps lessen skin irritation. Also be sure to put on a thick layer of a body butter or aloe vera–based moisturizer before you return to your day.

If you're like me and can't wax (no matter the cold or hot or microwave "easy" formula), try Sally Hansen's Spa Gel Hair Remover. It leaves skin smooth, and the dewy, hairless feel you have afterward will be especially appreciated by a woman who also goes for a "Brazilian." Put the gel on heavy for best results; it won't drip.

BEAM IT AWAY The newest way to remove unwanted hair is the most expensive. However, it is painless and very long-lived compared with electrolysis, which has been, up until now, the only potential form of permanent hair removal but is slow and painful. The new lasers can smite hair off our legs and bikini area almost permanently. Counting the product that ends up on the floor and the stuff needed to relieve the itch after, you can spend real money on your depilatory, so laser may not ultimately be as expensive as it seems. Has laser hair removal been around long enough for you to trust it? You'd never know it from all the hair removal home kits, electrolysis ads, and products out there, but it has!

You'll want to check out price, effectiveness, trouble, risks, and recovery time when considering any medical procedure. First off, how long will it last? The effects of the treatments will last for years; at the most you'll have to have a touch-up in the remote future. Second, who does it? Laser hair removal requires a state license. You can choose from a doctor whose treatments include it, or a salon or specialty parlor. There may be a new laser center in your area to check out.

Although it seems as if our hair is always growing, hair actually has active and rest phases. Once the rest phase is over, the strand falls out and a new one begins to grow. With laser removal, the hair can be removed only in the growth phase, when the cells at the base of the follicle divide and form new hair, which is pushed out onto the skin surface. The melanin pigment in the hair absorbs the laser light; then the light is converted to heat energy, which rapidly heats the hair all the way down to the follicle, effectively destroying the hair follicle. The hair ceases to grow while the surrounding skin and tissue are spared. Unfortunately, if you have very blond hair, this method won't work because there's no pigment to absorb the laser light.

Since all the follicles are not active at the same time, laser hair removal requires multiple treatments. Approximately 20 percent of the hair on your legs is in the growing phase at any one time, so treatments over two to five months are required to remove all the unwanted hair.

No matter how you approach it, hair removal (including shaving) is really annoying and dull. To help you get through it, I offer this story of how portentous the whole matter was for an ancient queen.

Three thousand years ago, news circulated of the beauty and brilliance of the Queen of Sheba. Rumors about her crisscrossed with tales of King Solomon's glory. Sheba wanted to meet Solomon, and he dreamed of her. At last Solomon took the initiative and sent a colorful, crested messenger bird (the hoopoe, often trained in the Middle East to serve the role of carrier pigeon over great expanses of desert) to Ethiopia to spy on Sheba.

The hoopoe turned into an ambassador, who spurred the queen to make the long journey to Solomon's court. When the king heard she was coming, he began to obsess. (Think Internet dating.) Though everybody praised the queen, it was said she had the hairy legs of a mountain goat.

Solomon, ever inventive, prepared a trap to see what lay under Sheba's gowns. A polished tile courtyard of marble was constructed, which he ordered to be filled with water one inch deep. When Sheba entered with her entourage and gifts were exchanged, the crafty king saw up her skirts in the pool's reflection. Indeed, the beauty's legs were covered with hair!

Solomon delighted in the queen, however, and arranged for a certain sticky pitch to be brought from the mountains, which he gave her as a depilatory. It worked, the royal persons consummated their love, and Sheba went home pregnant and happy to rule her own kingdom and spawn the first king of a new, long-lived Ethiopian dynasty.

TANNING

Tanning salons use ultraviolet light, and ultraviolet light causes cancer. Going under the bulbs in a tanning booth may be okay if you are pursuing a healthy glow for a special occasion or a boost to your self-image, but don't do it as a regular course of action.

If your skin type is fair, you may think you really need a tan. To get that base tan will take four to six sessions, with several days between sessions. The professional at the tanning salon will ask you about how quickly you tan and burn to time the sessions appropriately. Don't expect an even toffee. Just as in the sun, you may tan fastest on your legs and/or burn on your neck; the fake sunshine may give spotty results. Your best bet at an even tan is to use a good suntan lotion and go for five or more sessions at the briefest recommended length of time.

Spray-on or airbrush tans are gaining popularity. If you choose this route you are definitely going to want a technician to do it for you. The spray-on tan is a liquid solution that combines aloe vera, a bronzer, and DHA (dihydroxyacetone), a chemical that interacts with the skin to burnish it over several hours. Treatments range from thirty dollars in a stand-up booth to five times that for a hand-applied tan.

Some doctors go easy on tanning salons, but most think they are a god-awful idea. As Dr. Ron Shelton of the New York Aesthetic Center says, "You are intentionally getting radiation and toxicity. That's what the brown color is on the skin, and ultraviolet A (UVA) is a cocarcinogen; it helps increase the chances of the ultraviolet B that you get, even on a cloudy day, creating problems in the future. Why pay someone money and undergo the risk of complications and looking older just to improve your appearance briefly?

"Ultraviolet A rays are the deepest penetrating rays. They weaken the support of the skin, both the collagen and the elastic fibers, and that's where the real photo damage comes from. Ninety percent-plus of the aged appearance is photo damage, not chronological aging."

The common ingredient in self-tanners is DHA. Cosmetic tanners containing this white crystalline powder have improved so much that if you put them on a small section at a time, you can get an even look. Tanning lotions also contain a buffer for the slightly acidic DHA. Some self-tanners are a bit gooey, so they will not spread easily. Before using a tanning lotion or cream, make sure it flows freely by testing it on the sole of your foot. You can get an even more uniform tan in a salon, where you are sprayed with minute particles using an airbrush.

Self-tanners are fine with Dr. Shelton. They are animal pigment that enters the dead layers of skin, which exfoliate within a week or two. But he urges that you not assume the color gives safety in the sun; you still need to wear sunscreen.

Skin is classified in six gradations, depending on how you tan and burn: Five and 6 are dark-skin groups, 4 always tans and never burns, 1s are those redheads and pale blondes who never tan. No matter what your skin type, sunscreen not only prevents tanning but also arrests the accelerated aging caused by sun exposure. It used to be thought that African-Americans lucked out with regard to damaging sun rays. However, it is now understood that a person with rich, dark skin can get broken veins, or brown or white spots from the same UVA or long ultraviolet rays that increase the risk of cancer in lighter-skinned people.

As you destroy your collagen with sun exposure, the supporting structure of the skin loosens up, dilates, and deteriorates. If you are outdoors between 10:00 A.M. and 4:00 P.M., you must wear sunscreen all over. Don't think your legs are immune. However, you don't have to use sunscreen when dashing outdoors at lunch or going for an early morning or late afternoon walk. The sunshine is less intense early and late in the day, and your legs simply won't mind.

But, the unseen UVB rays do something you're really not going to like if you are prone to spider veins. UVBs, the burning rays, cause the capillaries near the surface of your skin to dilate and carry more blood, creating heat and a red appearance. Get into the habit, when your legs are bare and you plan to walk outside for fifteen minutes or more, of putting on a light moisturizer in the morning that protects you from the rays.

Use a moisturizer with sunscreen, such as the Neutrogena, Clinique, Shiseido, or L'Oréal brands. These self-tanners will give an even "natural" look: St. Tropez, Sun Labs, Fake Bake, and Xen-Tan. Air Stocking Sheer Bronze Tinted Self Tanning for Legs, and Bloom's Aloha Body Shimmer Cream are two more very effective self-tanning creams. Be sure to combine use of a self-tanner with a body hydrator, such as Caudalie Grape-Seed Body Lotion, L'Occitane Shea Butter Body Lotion, or Bliss Silky Lemon Sage Silky Milk, since the tanner may dry your skin.

You have to be careful with tanning not to end up with scaly legs or prematurely aged skin, but you do want that bronzy glow. You can't show your legs without being tan! The whole "to be or not to be" tan issue was transformed by Coco Chanel. People used to think that only lowly workers were exposed to the sun; then Coco bared her legs on the French Riviera and a tan pair of gams became a symbol of affluence. We can't beat the way tan color is identified with luxurious, sexy legs, but we can and should get the tanning effect as safely as possible—sans salons.

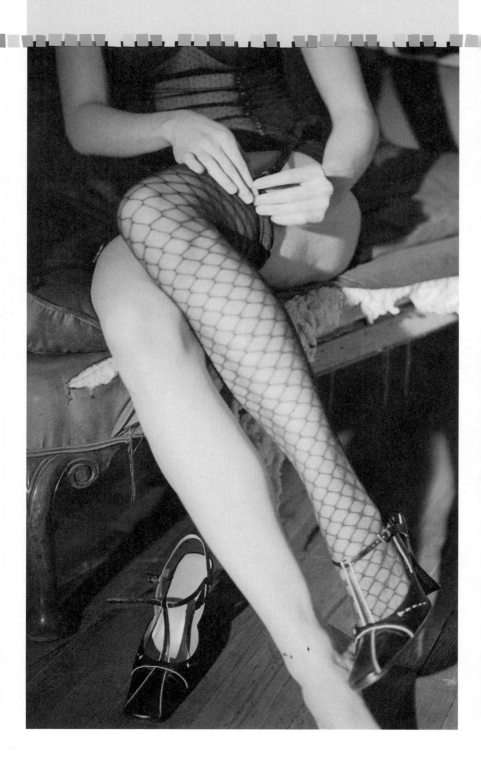

Dressing the Legs

TAKING STOCK

The lure of hose is timeless. From its beginning as linen leg coverings in ancient Greece and Rome, leg wear has evolved from tights to stockings and modern panty hose. Men originally wore the most ostentatious leg wear, and it took centuries for women's hosiery to become as decorative. In 1565 Queen Elizabeth's first pair of hand-knit silk hose was plain black. By the 1900s women's stockings were anything but boring, even though hemlines remained long. French stockings made from cotton, wool, or silk had elaborate designs, such as appliquéd snakes coiled around the entire leg. Other stockings featured wide embroidered appliqués with jewels and metallic thread that ran across the front leg.

The demand for stockings rose with hemlines in the 1920s, but solid colors—black, white, beige, and gray—were the most popular. When hemlines dropped in the 1930s, knee-high, flesh-toned stockings were in vogue, yet hosiery in films was far more exotic. In the 1935 film *The Devil Is a Woman*, Marlene Dietrich wore black stockings with a gold scalloped appliqué that ran from the tops of her feet to her thighs.

Once nylon stockings arrived, in 1940, women stood in line for hours waiting for hosiery departments to open. When fabric rationing put a hold on the production of nylons during

World War II, women artificially colored their legs with special cosmetics or used inexpensive products such as gravy browning or cocoa. Some women even painted seams up the backs of their calves to give the appearance of stockings. Marlene Dietrich painted her legs with gold metallic paint that closed her pores and made her collapse on the set of *Kismet* in 1944.

Nylon emerged again in the 1950s, when fabric rationing ended. Flesh or tan was the favorite color for most women, but black fishnet stockings ruled in films. During the 1960s and '70s, panty hose became a staple as hemlines rose. Seamless panty hose exploded in bright colors, geometric patterns, fishnets, and lace. Lycra was invented in 1959, but gained popularity during the 1960s and '70s. It was used in heavy denier tights. Kneesocks were also big and came in bright colors like "screaming pink," named after the film *Psycho.* Leg wear toned down several notches in the 1980s, when more neutral tones accompanied the "dress for success" fashion. Sheer legs knit with Lycra spandex revolutionized panty hose. Until then Lycra was primarily found in heavier tights, light support hose, and the control-top panty.

Today glitz is in for socks and panty hose. Since the 1990s panty hose and sock designs have reflected the styles of the 1960s and '70s. Socks come in bright citrus colors, muted pastels, stripes, polka dots, and flowers. Some are embellished with velvet rosettes, ribbons, or hand-crocheted bumblebees dangling off them.

The choices in panty hose are endless, including stockings in a bottle called Air Stockings, which give the illusion of stockings on bare legs. Panty hose come in a multitude of designs, including lace, with bands sewn around the legs, or embroidered polka dots. Seamed stockings are back, with herringbone or link-patterned seams. Catherine Zeta-Jones wearing cream-colored fishnet stockings in *Chicago* and Nicole Kidman in thigh-high, lace-topped, black stockings in *Moulin Rouge* inspired women to wear exotic hosiery with everyday fashion.

Women want to be sexy (sometimes), attractive (all the time), and comfortable (as much as possible). What Van Cleef & Arpels is to jewelry, Pratesi is to sheets, and Guerlain to perfume, Wolford is to hosiery. Since its founding in Austria in 1950, it has built an unequaled reputation for quality and design. The Wolford fabrics are light as air, energizing, velvety soft, and always practical and durable, not "disposable." No wonder, since they use yarn they invent—knockoffs are thus impossible. And it was in the ultrachic Wolford store in Soho in New York City that the world of hosiery, its traditions and its fads, was illuminated by Kymberlee Harris, Wolford's public relations person for the USA. It's what's underneath that counts, and European women have always looked to Wolford lingerie as the ultimate accessory.

JANE: **What is currently sexy in hose, in a broad sense?**
KYMBERLEE: This is such a personal thing, but for Wolford, being that we are produced in Austria, there is a certain conservativeness to many of the designs, but always a collection of the attention grabbers that many would find sexy. Wolford has a way of creating designs with opaque and transparent interplay, so that parts are covered and others revealed discreetly, such as bands of opaque material or squares.

JANE: **What's the difference between a fashion statement and sexy?**
KYMBERLEE: People with real style can wear anything, and if they exude confidence about themselves, they are also sexy! Because confidence is attractive, and everyone wants that. Luckily, wearing an interesting design on the legs can make a real statement. I get looks from both men and women even wearing a simple pattern on the legs, and people seem to enjoy seeing it. I even have young urban-type messengers very politely say to me, "Nice stockings," which I find surprising.

JANE: **There's an antihose movement, bare even in winter, bare with sandals.**

KYMBERLEE: Sad but true—it's my daily battle! It's all the fault of the fashion editors touting leg wear as "in" but showing bare legs with furs, gloves, and the whole nine. This looks ridiculous and unfinished and cold in the winter! Unless you have a gorgeous year-round tan, it does not look attractive on pasty white, goose-bumpy skin! It's shocking people don't realize this, even just for comfort's sake. Comfort is so important to us in this era, but I have been told that it's a luxury not to have to wear hosiery and to have a sedan waiting to sweep you away so you don't get cold in the winter. That is not the life of the norm, though, so only the super-rich and models should even attempt this look.

JANE: **Can hose make my legs look better?**

KYMBERLEE: Absolutely. We make supersheer nudes that you cannot even see. It's what we call "foundation for the skin." It covers imperfections and smoothes the coloring for an even look, and can even be slimming with a subtle shimmer. We like to think of our products as second skin.

JANE: **What can you wear instead of panty hose if you hate the way they go on and how they make you feel fat?**

KYMBERLEE: Funny enough, I don't like to wear nylons, but I do love the fishnets/ajourés (lattice knits) and opaques because they feel so soft. They move with your body and don't make you feel stuffed in like a sausage.

JANE: **Is there a support hose that looks sexy and mimics sheer?**

KYMBERLEE: We have a very special item called Invisible 12, and it is very sheer with an invisible "girdle area." It looks like a regular sheer nylon but holds you in. We also have thicker tights that shape and form your body. Some push up your butt or keep your legs energized with graduated knitting for better circulation points.

JANE: I would love to wear hose with the short skirts that are my sort of Betsey Johnson conceit, but they make my skirts ride up, so I don't.

KYMBERLEE: Overknee socks are good, or I just love the opaques (Velvet de Luxe 50). An old stylist trick I learned was using hair spray around the bottom of your skirt, which eliminates the static. Try it. We don't have any antistatic tights.

JANE: Does anybody normal buy garters?

KYMBERLEE: We got a lot of fashion editorials touting the garter and stockings. It is a small portion of our business, but our special, more elaborate sets do the best and make great gifts. I think they are more for special occasions.

JANE: What are the stay-ups about? (I mean stockings that aren't suspended.)

KYMBERLEE: Stay-ups are stockings with silicone bands to keep them on your legs. They are great, especially with fishnets, which can be tricky getting up and down for trips to the bathroom all day. They are great in the summer and just give you more freedom. Some people wear only the stay-ups and love them. I'm not fat, but I do get paranoid about bulges, so I prefer the tights.

JANE: What is there in Wolford's marvelous array in the range of tinted pastel hose, sparkly hose, hose with fake jewels, fishnets, and such?

KYMBERLEE: We pride ourselves on "novelties." We also have something special for holidays and do shimmers or metallics. We don't do too many pastels but do have a soft pink that is a classic in the collection (always available). We have a tight with randomly placed crystals that is divine! It comes in black or nude. I think the nude with crystal is gorgeous.

JANE: There are sometimes hose fashions, like the Cat in the Hat, that aren't sexy or particularly attractive but are fun.

KYMBERLEE: You can put on a plain black dress and crazy tights and you will get a conversation going in that outfit alone. I'm not kidding.

JANE: **Is there—maybe a very costly panty hose—that doesn't constrict?**
KYMBERLEE: Gosh, our tights never constrict. Controls are stiff, but if you try an opaque tight you will feel complete freedom of movement. It doesn't cost more. Getting the right size and fit is the key. Our sales people are so good about making sure the fit is right.

JANE: **That line down the back—does it come and go as a fashion?**
KYMBERLEE: It became a classic in the collection, and the fashion designers love it. Lagerfeld uses it even with his initials. We did a collaboration with Giorgio Armani but only through wholesale accounts, and he uses a back seam on nearly every style, so I would say it's very important at the moment. I think it is part of the pencil skirt, chic secretary look that is in fashion now, but it could fade away eventually.

JANE: **Now, tell me what men like to buy for women when they come in without their wives and girlfriends.**
KYMBERLEE: The lingerie sets, for sure! They might not know the size but can guess from looking at other women, and things can be exchanged.

JANE: **Any stars and celebrities you can mention whom I'll meet stopping by the Soho store?**
KYMBERLEE: So many! To name a few, Sharon Stone, Mary J. Blige, Shannen Doherty, Elizabeth Hurley, Annette Bening, Catherine Zeta-Jones, Elaine Stritch, Marie Osmond, Stephanie Seymour, Katie Couric, Oprah, Linda Evangelista, Kirsten Dunst, Amber Valletta, et cetera.

Great Legs!

In general, my attitude is, Who would want the hassles of being rich? I get it once in a while, though, like when I put on very fine hose and feel the difference all day long. Wolford is the number one line because it's durable and well-constructed, but Soleil Toile, the lovely big lingerie store in my town, says only good things about the number two line, Donna Karan, as well. Says the manager, Pam Como, "Currently nude is the way to go, and from Donna Karan comes a variety of nudes: The degrees are defined by numbers, so you can match your own skin tone. You choose from sheer, control, or longer control 'essential toner.'"

You don't need to wipe out your whole bin of stockings to get one marvelous pair. If you do, put them in the lingerie bag before you cold wash in the machine. If you hand wash, there is an especially good product called Forever New, for hose and other fragile fabrics.

Sometimes you want a good line without the stocking look. Spanx go down to the knee or all the way down to the ankle and are footless hose.

Soleil Toile advises that white or ecru hose are purely for weddings. (Evidently the pairs of petal pink and white stockings in my drawer have to wait out the present minimalism in hose, or be refashioned as Barbie outfits.)

All legs are not created equal, yet every leg can appear longer, sleeker, smoother, or shapelier with a few fashion and cosmetic tricks. With some ingenuity and creativity, even the most problem legs can be a fashion asset. Think of your legs as an accessory that belongs with your outfits.

Start with the basics. To elongate shorter legs, wear monochromatic outfits, such as black stockings, black skirt, and a black top. Wearing a different color on top will make you and your legs look shorter. Longer legs can afford to be seen in print skirts and solid tops, but stay away from head-to-toe patterns.

Calves deserve special attention, and the length of skirt can enhance or detract from their shape. For skinny calves, be sure to focus on lighter-colored stockings; fishnets or patterned tights will make them seem larger. Also, wearing skirts at or slightly above the knee is most flattering. Avoid dark stockings and miniskirts so your legs will not look like poles. Larger calves, by contrast, look best in darker solid-color stockings or tights, and skirts are best worn midcalf or at the knee, with a straighter cut. Full skirts or pleats merely add to the apparent size of heavier legs.

Shoes can also change the look of calves and ankles. High heels elongate the calf, while flat shoes make calves appear larger. Medium heels look best on most legs. Thin ankles look great with ankle-strap shoes or sandals, but thick ankles are not flattered by ankle straps or thick wedge soles.

Bare legs are in, and cosmetic touches should never be lost on legs. Make up your legs as you would your face, with a bronzer or spray-on stocking to hide imperfections and give the illusion of flawless skin.

Finally, remember that pants are problem legs' best friends and can play up a shapely bottom or hide scrawny calves. Even if you were not blessed with a "bubble" bottom, you can simulate the tight curve in the new ultrachic cotton-Lycra jeans, which act as girdles to smooth lumpy thighs and derrieres. Stick with darker blues for a slimmer look. Of course, black pants are timeless and look great on just about anyone's legs. Try on the very expensive black pants of ethereal fabrics before you settle for a bargain; black pants are a fashion item where a bit more money is well spent.

Mary Lou's
BEADED ANKLET 101

MATERIALS LIST:
- 1 clasp, spring form, and jump ring
- 2 bead tips
- Beading thread, Nymo, or heavy upholstery thread
- Beading needle, small enough to go through the beads with thread
- Jeweler's glue
- Round-nose pliers, small enough to fit in the bead tip
- Assortment of small glass or metal beads (not seed beads); keep the beads small so they don't interfere with your leg resting on furniture

INSTRUCTIONS:

First, measure your ankle to determine how long you are going to make your anklet, leaving room so it can move about on your leg.

Thread your beading needle with a double length of Nymo or thread at least 36 inches long. On the loose end, tie on a bead small enough to fit inside the bead tip. A few overhand knots will work. Add the bead tip so that it covers the bead and so the hook end is going to the outside. Now it is time to start beading. Add the beads in the order you desire, either in a pattern or random.

When you have a string of beads about 2 inches shorter than your desired length, stop and add the other bead tip, with the hook going inside. Now add 1 tiny bead. Take your needle and go under the bead and out the top to create a loop around the bead. You are doing this to create a tighter knot.

Cut your thread from the needle, leaving enough thread to work with. Pull the threads tight but not too tight, just enough to take out any slack. Tie a couple of square knots: left over right and right over left. You are almost done! Add a spot of glue in each of the bead tips, and close the tips with your pliers. Now attach the clasp by closing the hook of each bead tip around the clasp. Congratulations, you now have a wonderful new anklet!

We don't have to wear stockings anymore because they are de rigueur at the workplace or a must with Sunday best. Hosiery is now elective and has emerged from being a practical part of attire to offering many possibilities to show off a pretty set of legs. Patterned tights can jazz up a miniskirt, dark sheer stockings will lengthen the line of the body, and funky socks identify one's sense of color and style.

Don't settle for any hosiery that is less than completely comfortable. The stockings or tights should move with ease. You want to wiggle your toes in socks that breathe and don't leave elastic marks. Try socks with sandals and bodysuits with slinky outfits. Buy hose at the pharmacy only in an emergency. Pass on a bargain six-pack of socks and buy the pair of running socks that match your activity. Look for a pair of happy, original, fashionable socks instead of those plain solids.

Women who pay attention to their clothes to please men and themselves do well not to forget to dress up their legs. Hosiery is a relatively inexpensive article of dress, yet it draws men's eyes to what most men view as our most beguiling female asset. Today's stretchy, silky weaves and array of colors and designs can actually make choosing stockings and socks entertaining. Go for this new frontier of self-expression and delight yourself and everybody else!

BODY DECOR

From Morocco to India, women put the markings of mehndi on their hands and feet as decoration for an auspicious occasion like a wedding. Berber women do it to ward off evil spirits. Certain Jewish women do it at a woman's bridal party. In Rajasthan, India, women lovingly decorate their bodies to prepare for a husband's return. The meaning is personal—"I feel special"—it has no ritual significance.

This is perhaps the oldest women's visual art form, done for thousands of years. Now it's sprung into a new fashion in Europe and the United States, especially where people have settled from India. Mehndi is the painting of patterns on the body using dried, powdered henna leaves. The patterns are very elaborate, and the color soft and flattering to skin tones. Since henna has medicinal properties, the henna painting conditions the skin as well. Mehndi actually refers to the oil the fine powder is mixed with, but you can also use eucalyptus oil. It commonly takes up to five hours to apply the dye. The mehndi lasts for several weeks, gradually fading from the original red, gray, or brown, the way autumn leaves do.

Henna painting is much easier to do today, and takes much less time, because instead of being applied with a stick of ivory or sandalwood, a paste is available in a nozzled tube. You can buy this online or at Indian stores, like the New York Body Archive, 9 Ninth Avenue, NY, NY 10011. Their henna kit sells for about twenty-five dollars and comes with the paste, instructions, and design sheets. You can also get mehndi at Indian bazaars and fund-raisers or at Indo-American organizations all over the United States.

Tattoos are another popular form of body art. When they see a tattoo on a woman, men either light up or turn off. There doesn't seem to be a middle ground. If a man likes to see a display of permanent art on a female ankle, it's because he's imagining the matching design somewhere else on her body.

Josh Glasser, a tattoo artist who owns Ink-Side-Out in downtown Norwalk, Connecticut, brings in major female clientele. "Women," says Josh, "lean to meaningful, colorful tattoos. Guys say, 'Give me a tiger on my back, or a Grim Reaper on my arm.' Women go more with meaning and aesthetics, and how it looks on their body." The most popular motifs are butterflies, small birds, flowers, especially roses, Chinese characters, and zodiac signs. Josh also has many requests for angels, roses, or hearts with a child's name. The symbol should reflect you.

After ankles and the bikini area, feet have become popular to decorate as well—in Josh's view "because it's the most rebellious." A smaller design takes twenty minutes. People say the pain is less than they expected. It just depends on your tolerance. The other factor is whether the tattoo will be on, for instance, the calf, where you will feel it much less than, say, on the inner thigh.

Tattooing has come a long way. Shops respect their clients and use high standards of cleanliness and brand-new needles for each customer. People are highly unlikely to get HIV from a tattoo, but if the operation is slipshod, there is a real chance of hepatitis. Dr. Robert J. Terdiman, a cardiologist in New York, advises against tattoos because "any bloodborne invasion of the body can spread HIV," he explains. "If the person is careless about sterilizing the needle you can get hepatitis B, which will make you dreadfully sick, or hepatitis C or HIV, which you will have forever." So never get a tattoo on impulse, and make sure you go to someone locally who has a good reputation. If there is no such person available, hold the thought. Seek referrals from other women you know whose tattoos you admire. Once you have selected a reputable place, look over the shop with a keen eye. Make sure the examples they show you are their own up-to-date work. Then ask to see a state license.

A dress is a dress, but it's the detail of your attire that

shows distinction or sizzle. A lot of grown women today are looking chic with anklets and discreet tattoos. Good motivation for a tattoo is to express your free spirit, and an anklet draws attention to the foot or shoe. Be very careful, though, that it's decor, not branding. In a sophisticated circle, you may find the only acceptable decoration for the legs is a pair of stockings!

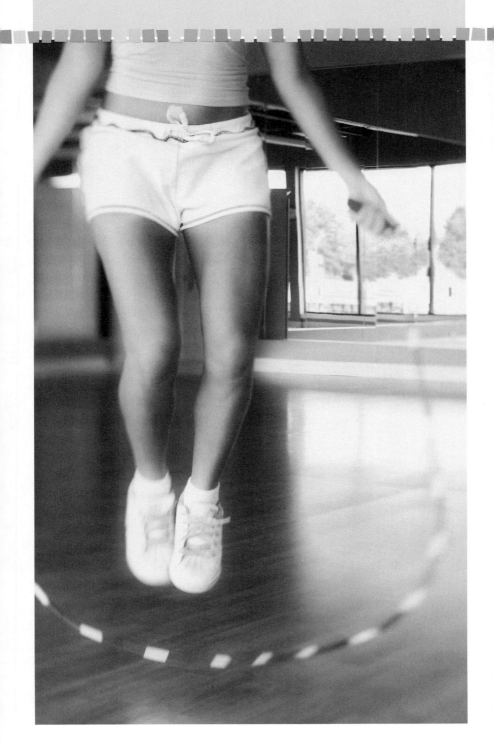

Exercises and Leg Awareness

FREUD SAID THAT anatomy is destiny. Today we like to take control of our destiny and improve on our anatomy. The happy news is that legs are the easiest part of your body to make attractive. You'll get beautiful leg tone and shape through pinpoint exercises and through whatever sport or physical activity you do. You can pretty much identify an athlete's chosen sport by the musculature, movement, and build of his or her body. Certain sports will give your legs a certain physicality and attractive look. If you want that look, take a class. You don't have to be a champion to have your legs benefit from exercise.

LEG EXERCISES

First of all, here are some important stretches that you should keep in mind before exercising, especially in the interest of achieving a greater range of motion.

BASIC LEG STRETCH (Passive.) Sit on the floor with your back straight, and spread your legs in front of you. Now spread them a little more. Curve your right arm over your head toward the left leg, bending at the waist. Inhale. As you exhale, move your arm all the way over the leg. Your head and torso remain facing forward. Reverse arms and repeat the stretch on the other side.

OVERHEAD STRETCH (Passive.) Lie flat on your back with your arms at your sides. Raise your legs over your head to a shoulder stand (but go only as far as comfortable). Support your lower back with your hands and hold your legs straight up for 5 breaths. Then move one leg overhead back toward the floor. Bring that leg back to the original position, then repeat with the other leg. Make the same movement using both legs together as you fold at the hips. Hold for 5 breaths. Bring the legs back up, then lower your back slowly, vertebra by vertebra, to the floor. This exercise brings blood back to the heart from the legs.

SLEEP EXERCISE (Passive.) No kidding, after this splendid exercise you can fall asleep! This works your thighs and primps your posture. Do this on your bed if the mattress is hard, or on a mat on the floor. Close your eyes. Lie on your left side. Breathe in and out a few times. Your left leg is bent slightly at the knee. Take the right leg and raise it over the left. Put the right heel on the left knee. Put your right arm behind you, expanding your chest and pulling up so you arch your torso. Repeat on the other side. Now rest or sleep.

Your legs are different from any other part of your body. If you walk a lot, they may get plenty of exercise without getting the range of motion that will make them truly strong and shapely. If you do a few exercises to hit calves and thighs, you will be amazed at how wrong Freud was that anatomy is determinate. Here are a traditional hula exercise (passive) that's a wake-up call to the upper legs, plus my mother's exercises to "slenderize" (sorry, that was her term) passively in a chair or your own bed. Lin Yutang said, "It is amazing how few people are conscious of the importance of the art of lying in bed." Now there are practitioners of lymphatic massage that will do this for you, but I think you can do it for yourself.

HULA EXERCISE This exercise, the Rainbow Arch, can

be done with a ball or without, on your own or with someone to "spot" you.

Lie back with your hips on the top of the ball. Plant your feet in line with your shoulders. Place your hands at either side of your head. Arch and stretch back. Curve as far as is comfortable, adjusting the spread of your legs for balance. Then release the ball and do this on the floor from the kneeling position. Think of stretching from the trunk and front of your body as, with hands behind your head, you gently fall back, curving from your hips.

If you have someone to help you, you can curve back farther. Done correctly, this exercise does not cause back strain. It is marvelous for your hip flexors, which are key to the hula and which get tight in adults. The trainer who incorporates hula exercises says, "The bigger the stretch, the bigger the gait: It's almost an antiaging drug."

MOM'S BED EXERCISE (Passive.) Sit on the floor with your knees scrunched up and legs bare. You're going to clasp and pinch the fleshier parts of your legs with your palms. Do it rapidly, don't hold. If this hurts, your body is tensing. The more pleasant the sensation the better the toxins are being flushed and fat dislodged from the cells. Travel up and down the hinges of your legs to your feet, on all sides. Then repeat, this time rolling the muscles between your flat hands. For example, if your left hand is pressing and pushing on top of your thigh, your right hand should be under the thigh moving in the other direction. This movement will be unfamiliar, but it effectively aids diet in whittling off undesired fat and toning loose areas.

Several other forms of exercise are good for shaping the legs. *Swimming* tones legs so well that you can see results in a month from just 45 minutes 5 days a week. Do some lengths of breaststroke for the thighs. Add high-impact exercise like *jumping rope* to make it a full hour; this is the perfect combo. If you enjoy water aerobics, you're going to have to have consummate form to get results, as this is a low-intensity approach. *Cycling* is a fast way to get muscle tone in the legs. You can supplement it with a brief routine of yoga, Pilates, or other stretches.

Running is a sustained, longer activity. Some athletes do warm-ups, but I don't like them. If I allot 60 minutes a day to exercising, I prefer to get right into it. Additionally, the Centers for Disease Control has concluded, "There is not sufficient evidence to endorse or discontinue routine pre-run or post-run stretching to prevent injury among competitive or recreational athletes." You can build up your running from less to more strenuous, slow to more rapid, and so forth. If you can run a mile, you can run eight miles (should you wish), if you pace yourself.

Establishing a route on which you run, walk, or bike intensifies the pleasure. It makes you more aware of life around you, and your pace. You come to possess the route; it becomes you, which is the secret to being consistent about your aerobic exercise. Ion Grumeza, trainer of gymnastics and weight lifting at the YMCA of Westport, Connecticut, emphasizes that rule number one is "Do not get hurt, and stop at any pain."

You tire less, sleep better, and have a more natural self-regulated appetite when you give your legs good use. What you do is mechanical, but the benefit is pervasive. Most important to me is mood. If you have a good temperament, you'll be positively radiant and serene if you do regular aerobic exercise. If you are under unusual stress, exercise will help you bear the stress more lightly. You can start small, by doing jumping jacks and squats, and work your way up to a run. You will gain energy. Do exercises to get gorgeous legs, but know that you'll gain a more positive mind-set as well. Here are some other exercises you might incorporate into your run.

MARIONETTE JUMPS (Active.) These are just great for the legs. Jump, swinging one leg to the side and return it to center. Then do the other leg, then alternate, shifting your center point as you move in the direction you are running. Do this for the length of a football field or whatever is comfortable. Relax your shoulders, arms, and hands so they flow like a bird's wings. Cross your arms in front of you for momentum.

BACK KICKS (Active.) The next variation is a modification of dancers' leaps. In a gentle run, let your fifth step be a leap. Rather than step with your next foot, kick that leg back and then glide it forward so you land as you would have without the kick. What matters is not how high you leap but getting a rhythm in which you feel a continuity of movement from your hips to the balls of your feet. With active back kicks, a run becomes a total leg workout.

INCLINE PUSH-UPS (Active.) Somewhere along your running route is a bicycle rack or railing three to four feet tall. Lower your body and then shoot back up to do incline push-ups. Full push-ups are the world's best overall exercise if you can do a lot of them, but these standing incline push-ups actually work the front thigh muscles better. Keep your body straight and go slowly so you feel you're working the upper thigh muscles.

The top exercise picks for fast leg results are spinning, in-line skating, ice skating, dancing, and fencing. The top picks to show off your legs are in-line skating, running, fencing, and coed volleyball. Putting the treadmill at a steeper incline, even one or two notches, will help build your calves in only six weeks!

When our lives are full and we don't have time to go to the gym, we can do passive exercises or exercises that fit into our normal activity. I suggest ankle weights for taking no time at all. Simple ankle weights are sold in sporting goods stores or on the Internet. Get a set of two-pound weights and Altus adjustable weights. The heavier weight is for more stationary work; the lighter for fast walking—or chasing the kids. You can incorporate these into your daily routine, and you'll be astonished how they develop the shapeliness of your calves and ankles.

There are numerous systems of exercise to choose from. All you need is one that's intelligent and effective for you. By that I mean you will *do* it, and do it without cheating. No matter what exercise you choose, you'll make it yours—by doing it at a certain time, on a certain day, or in a certain place.

No matter which way you improve your legs through exercise, from time to time you need to shore up what you do. For this I recommend yoga. Many yoga videotapes or DVDs are good, or take a class if you have time. In all types of yoga, concentration makes you aware of the fronts, backs, and sides of your legs, so you internalize your condition as you gradually improve it.

Yoga is a multivalent exercise that is good for the whole core of your body. It looks pretty if you're in company and can be done while you're home talking on the phone. Extend your right leg behind you as you lean forward, and grab your right ankle with your right hand. Now think of yourself as a hood ornament on a vintage Packard and you'll get it right.

Between ages twenty and forty, your total muscle mass can decrease up to 40 percent, yet there is evidence that with proper attention to exercise you can restore it, and be just as strong at eighty. Slow Burn Fitness is an inspiring plan to reverse the loss of strength that comes with age. The focus is not only to increase muscular strength but to benefit other body systems, especially the heart and lungs. Fredrick Hahn, the guru of Slow Burn Fitness, says, "Slow Burn turns the body into a fat-burning machine." Fred suggests the heel raise as one of his exercises that you can do at home to get shapely calves fast. Once you see the results, you might want to enter more deeply into the Slow Burn program, using Fred Hahn's *Slow Burn Fitness Revolution* (Broadway Books, 2003), which is especially good for people with fraught schedules and high fitness goals.

FRED HAHN'S HEEL RAISE Grab two towels and set your timer for 100 seconds. Roll the towels and place them side by side horizontally 3 feet from a wall. Step onto the towels, with the ball of each foot at the center of a towel. Place your hands directly in front on you on the wall, and lock the position. Lean forward slightly by bending your elbows. Rise onto your toes and the balls of your feet 1 inch per second. Pause to squeeze your calf muscles in both legs, then reverse and lower. It's 7 seconds up, 7 down. Your heels should scarcely touch the floor before you slowly rise again.

Rowers do a number of leg exercises, the most popular of which is called Jumpies. This involves squatting to the ground by bending your knees while extending your arms straight out in front of you, then jumping up as high as you can while throwing your arms for propulsion. This exercise gives legs a great workout, and any number of Jumpies is helpful for developing muscle mass.

I think of my exercises as a recipe box. So many have nice associations of where and how I learned them. My souped up sit-ups, for instance, were demonstrated (and named) by a very handsome parachutist named Louis, who explained that parachutists have to develop their leg muscles. Do a dozen each of these and you'll feel you've accomplished great things!

SOUPED-UP FULL SIT-UP WITH BALL (Active.) Using a soccer or kids' ball or a three- to four-pound medicine ball at the gym, hold the ball over your head as you lie on your back, and bring the ball over your head and forward as you move into the sit-up.

SOUPED-UP SCISSOR SIT-UP (Active.) Begin by lying on your back. Place your arms straight out over your body. As you rise and push forward, spread your legs and position your head and arms in one plane the way a diver would. Tense, hold, and try to move forward to do the best sit-up you can. Then close your legs as you return to the original lying down position.

You can't address your whole being at once. You have to

latch on to parts of it at a time. If you focus on one body part, it will affect your posture. You can use this knowledge to prevent fatigue as well as to "sculpt" your legs. For example, if you run and your legs start to ache, focus on raising your breasts. As you do, you'll notice the weight and force in your legs are distributed differently. This simple change in orientation can allow you to run more miles when you would otherwise be tired. Focused exercises such as the scissors sit-ups will oxygenate your legs and increase blood flow. You will have more energy and reserve it better. You will lose excess weight in the pinpointed area so it is more attractive. Difficult, focused exercise is well worth it, because it will bring invaluable toning to your body. Before doing several vigorous sets of any strenuous exercise, consult with your doctor or fitness specialist.

I am a proponent of having fun doing exercise, without stopwatches or much technical knowledge. You don't have to know a quad from a glute to transform your thighs, but you do have to think very three-dimensionally. Consider a thigh as having a top, with which you are well-acquainted, an underside you spy when you try on bathing suits, and outer and inner sides. Any exercise in which you *feel it* will register improvement, so first of all notice when you ache. Thighs can ache from biking, fencing, dance, or sex, and that's clearly a good thing. At the gym there are machines that address the parts I've just mentioned using the unattractive-sounding words glutes (buttocks), quadriceps (front thighs), hamstrings (back thighs), abductors (outer thighs) and adductors (inner thighs). You can tone and whittle your thighs out on those machines. However, to make the biggest difference in the shortest time, you need to address your thigh issues yourself every day in every way. The most basic ways are ball work and Pilates. You need a ball, a mat, a video or DVD or two, and ten thigh-focus minutes in the morning and later in the day.

Ball work is fun and has multiple benefits. It also works the midsection of your body when you are doing an exercise specific to the legs. You can try out the different-sized balls at your sports store.

(1) Seated on the ball with your feet flat on the floor, the angle formed by your hips and knees should be 90 degrees. Or go by this rule of thumb: If you are four foot eleven to five foot four, you need a 21-inch (53 centimeter) size, whereas if you are five feet or over, the best size is 25 inches (65 centimeters). Go bigger if you are heavy and smaller if you are lightweight. Don't fully inflate the ball the first time you use it; it's easier to do these exercises better when the ball is underinflated because less balancing is required.

After you do this short ball workout, pick up the ball and hold it over your head. (2) Standing tall, roll your wrists so that the ball nods forward and backward. A few inches back, and forward all the way to your knees, or just a few inches; alternate. Raise the ball over your head and dip it with a gliding motion to the right and then the left.

About half the women I know thicken at the waist; the other portion of us thicken at the thighs, inner and/or outer. Pilates is the answer, but you don't have to get into the inner sanctum of yet another exercise program to reap its benefits. You can get as deep as you need from a simple video or DVD. Using movements on a mat, Pilates includes an intensive core routine. You practice breathing as well, so you can push yourself with the contractions and not get fatigued.

Pilates can be done with or without a ball, on your own, or with someone to "spot" you. (3) Begin with the Rainbow Arch exercise mentioned earlier. Lie back on your hips on top of the ball. Plant your feet in a line with your shoulders. Place your hands at either side of your head. Arch and stretch back. Curve back as far as is comfortable, adjusting the spread of your legs for balance.

Next, release the ball and do the exercise on the floor from a kneeling position. (Or start from this position.) Think of stretching from your front trunk. With hands behind your head, gently lean back, curving from your hips. If you have someone to help, you can curve even farther back. Done correctly this does not cause back strain. This stretch is marvelous for your hip flexors, which can get tight in adults.

(4) The Prone Circus Poodle Level One (active) is another exercise to try. Start by lying on the ball facedown. Position the ball so it supports your torso. Roll forward until your hands are on the floor. Roll back and forth, and as you do, raise your legs. Repeat 5 times. Next, repeat the same motion but raise your right leg and left arm at the same time. Alternate by raising your left leg and right arm. Do 5 times. Additional exercises will be included with your ball.

After you gain some skill in using the ball, try my favorite for your legs. Level Two: Same prone starting position, but this time bring your thighs up on the ball into a crouching position. Rest there like a human paperweight or your own circus act! Balance and return to the prone position. Repeat 5 or more times. Level Three is doing this same crouch but with no hands!

If your legs are too skinny, you'll want to build them up with exercise. Skinny legs can become varicose legs if you get even thinner and the muscles break down. Also, cold temperatures can hinder your circulation if you have scant flesh on your bones. As a result, your veins become more brittle, and that's not good.

Strong is what you want. Upper and lower legs are beautiful that work out and work. If you think your legs lack contour, do some calf exercises. In addition, you can smear a bit of body shimmer on your legs to highlight the contours you've got.

Of all the approaches to exercising your legs, in terms of beauty, the smartest is to add a little athleticism to your movements throughout the day. If you lengthen your gait, use perfect posture, and lift and stretch as you move, if you climb stairs and dance doing chores around the house, you are exercising without having to look at the clock in the gym. Whatever exercise form you choose, make sure you feel the opposition from the muscles to know it's having the beautifying effect.

PRAISE YOUR LEGS ROUTINE

Do you feel affection for or disaffection for your legs? Wear sweatpants all the time and your legs lose some shape. Run in cute shorts and your legs look more youthful. It does seem to matter. If your legs feel blah and you take them for granted, they lose tone. If you have an overbearing or mechanistic attitude toward your legs, or a perfectionist, frustrated attitude, they will be less beautiful. If you have a positive vantage, your legs will dance their way through the day. Dr. Andrew Gentile, a practicing clinical psychologist, states, "Focusing on your legs can be an effective way to create beautiful legs." If you pay attention to some aspect of your legs that you like, your increased awareness can lead to actions that will bring about change. These positive results will in turn give you the confidence to make even greater changes. Rather than ruminate about how bad your legs look, measure small positive changes that are taking place. In this way, you are shifting your attention from a negative outcome to a positive process. Focus on the positive because doing so leads to positive action, self-confidence, and eventual change.

All the research on mind-body says that we change our bodies through our thoughts. Only looking, however, isn't enough. Just paying attention creates negative and positive feedback, so you have to focus on what the legs are: assets. Look not at the outcome of a beauty program but at the positive process. Here is a weekly routine.

MONDAY:

SET YOUR MIND Use simple biofeedback. Watch a sports event with women athletes on television. See a movie with legs to admire, such as *Silk Stockings, South Pacific,* or *Bend It Like Beckham.* When you notice great legs, think, "My legs are terrific."

TUESDAY:

PRAISE YOUR LEGS Think of what they have accomplished. You walked up the Arc de Triomphe or stayed up on water skis the first time out. As you focus on your legs, think, "You did great." This may feel weird, but it is just like the gardener who talks to her flowers.

WEDNESDAY:

LOOK AT YOUR LEGS As you walk past store windows, or exercise in the gym, look at your gams. You look into long mirrors often, but this is seeing yourself in motion. Feel good to be alive. Step up the movement so you move with more lift, and look again.

THURSDAY:

LIE DOWN AND MOISTURIZE YOUR LEGS Then do sexy bicycles and lifts. Point your toes and think how sexy your legs are when they're in the mood.

FRIDAY:

DO SOMETHING PLAYFUL WITH YOUR LEGS Remember yourself as a girl using your legs in an equally playful way. It could be jumping rope, doing jumping jacks, leaping, or sitting on a table swinging your legs. This is an exercise not to exert you but to reorient you—unclench the gravity—and your adult feelings.

SATURDAY AND SUNDAY:

TAKE A WALK AND THINK, "I am renewing my legs. They are becoming prettier, longer, and stronger."

Great Legs!

POSTURE AND SEX APPEAL

With women's liberation, it became fashionable to show off a fit female body. But sometimes there's an attitude of "I look good, but if you undress me with your eyes, I'll slap you with a sexual harassment suit." Marilyn Monroe's sex appeal predated the feminist movement and made men of the caliber of Joe DiMaggio and Arthur Miller marry her. It's often pointed out that she was heavier than the present standard of gorgeous. Since she is in all our minds, it's just a half step more to think what she did that we can adapt for those days when we want to be a bit more sexy than ordinary.

Marilyn had an energy field. She kept it in place. She was relaxed, yet she kept her chest high and her pelvis tilted back—ideal for beauty and health. When she stood or walked, she always added a grace note. That's the lesson in watching her move. She would tense slightly from stasis. If sitting, she would sit and then move forward in the chair and lift. If standing, she would twist a beat after she came to the standing position, or tense her thighs. These were very small movements that added sizzle to her poses. Try it in a mirror. This is a primitive yet natural sexing up of your posture.

Basically, we're talking about posture and pose. Again, it's tip up, twist, and swish. Here are a few poses that will make any woman project her demure body flirtation.

I went to a prep school that practically invented the debutante slouch. My mother despaired over that slouch and had me walk with a book on my head. This was dangerous for my terrier, Queenie, who followed me wagging her tail, so my mother came up with something that worked—the plumb line. Imagine a string attached to the top of your head that suspends you. As it is pulled, you feel your body grow taller and your spinal cord lengthen. Your chest rises, and your fanny goes where it belongs, behind, not under the hips.

For alignment and beautiful posture, your legs are essential.

Posture is the most important element of your body's attractiveness, and the only one you can change relatively quickly. Just dedicating an extra moment to adjust your posture can make all the difference. When sitting in a chair, cross one leg over the other on top of the lower knee and point your foot. Never be frontal with your body when you are observed. When standing in line, advance one leg slightly to the side of the other. When the right leads, it angles left; when the left leads, it angles right. If you are seated on a hassock or low bench, stretch your feet and legs out and cross your ankles. Stretching is key.

Notice how female Olympic medalists with the most stunning lines to their legs and posture are those who do the 100-meter dash, hurdles, and long jump, where posture is central. I have also seen the best posture in women in the fields of India and western Asia who carry baskets and buckets on their heads.

THE ART OF
Matthew Barney

At the beginning of this millennium, the Guggenheim Museum in New York dedicated the entire exhibition space to a rare one-artist show. Every review said the original mythology and personal legend that the young American sculptor and painter Matthew Barney had created for the winding circular ascent of this museum was the most entrancing show in decades. All through the indescribable magical story were repeating themes. Recalling its beautiful, strong goddess legs, I asked Matthew Barney to reflect on what he sees in the leg from a sculptural perspective.

As a high school quarterback, I was taught to assume a position with my body where my legs were bent at the knee and where one foot would turn slightly inward with the heel elevated, while the other foot pointed straight ahead and remained flat on the ground. This was the basic stance I would take every time I put my hands under the center's butt. From this position, I could move laterally in either direction, and the in-turned foot would give me a half-step head start in a straight drop back. I always found this customized posture very elegant, both for its dynamic look and in the way that it harnessed and stored potential energy.

The aesthetics of this stance led me to a fixation on the form of the wedge (when I started making sculpture in college). The wedge was the first of a number of abstractions I started making when I began to call upon my past experiences as an athlete to construct an aesthetic system. The wedge could represent the negative space under my cleated right foot in the starting stance. As such, it could suggest the potential for movement, or action, when placed under an inanimate object.

As this aesthetic system began to grow, characters developed, along with a story line. While the stories were essentially ritualized conflicts (like football), the characters started becoming more and more diverse. There were male and female coded characters, all of which I would play. As I found myself in high-heeled shoes, I thought about some of those things I had imagined as a teenager. The way the wedge beneath my heel put my leg into tension, made me taut. At least formally, it appeared that I could spring from this position, suggested by the angle of my foot and the way it flexed every muscle in my lower leg. It felt that way, too—to be in a shoe of that shape for the first time—it felt like I had potential to explode, perhaps not laterally but definitely forward.

LEGS AND SEX

To a man, our legs denote unconsciously the path to glory. "You gaze at me teasingly through the window; a virgin face . . . and below . . . a woman's thighs." (Praxilla, fifth century B.C.)

When we are young to sex, our legs tremble. It's like the first time we go mountain hiking. When the unaccustomed movements grow more familiar, our legs grow stronger in them. A woman who has a caring partner unclenches in her mind; then she can express desire and rapture, silliness and laughter, and affection, all with the semaphoric language of her legs.

THIRTEEN WAYS THAT LEGS SAY LOVE

The role of our legs in sexual behavior is rarely given a second thought, yet from flirtation all the way to coitus they play a central role. The following thirteen points come from women who observed themselves or thought back over their love lives, to articulate what legs can accomplish in the flirty and passionate modes.

1. "YOU'RE MY MAN" (STANDING). Let's say you're standing waiting for a guy. At the same moment, he's approaching you for lunch, a date, or a serious encounter. Rather than face toward him or the direction from which he's coming, turn slightly and twist to the side. Create a tension in your hips. This tiny seductive movement says you relate to him as an attractive male without being in the least overt.

2. "YOU'RE MY MAN" (SEATED). If you are sitting (not sprawled) on a chair, respond to him by swiveling instead of turning. If you swivel to the right, bring your right leg fast against and slightly over your left. (Vice versa if he is to the left of you.) The swivel says you are accepting of him sexually, but drawing back your leg says you aren't too easy to get.

3. "I'M FEELING FLIRTY." On a date or if you are lounging with your mate, sit on the floor while relating to him, no matter where he sits. Legs plainly stretched is very matter-of-fact, while crossed legs suggest androgyny. Whether you take a modest or a saucy pose, point your feet a little and raise your torso. Your expression could be that of someone at a symphony hall, but the message conveyed awakens him.

4. "TRY ME." Extend the Golden Rule from the general to the particular. For him to discover the pleasure of stroking your legs may take your stroking his, from the inner thighs to the ankles and toes. In the communication that makes sex really interesting, we all mirror each other's moves. Discover his sensitive spots, whether behind his knees or above his ankles, to increase his awareness of being attracted to your gams.

5. "I'M READY." Since men are so visual, it does a couple great good for a man to have a big mental album of all the cute poses his woman takes in bed. The optimal moment is when you are in bed first. The idea is to be fetching: There's a pinup girl in each of us waiting to be discovered! Raising your knees to your chin and sitting over your legs with the right tucked over the left (chest held high) are turn-ons for a guy. Sitting primly like Red Riding Hood's grandmother, with legs clenched in front of you, a book, and cookies and ginger ale on the bed table is, conversely, a turnoff for most men, even if you're dressed in Frederick's of Hollywood!

6. "UNWRAP ME AND LET'S DO IT!" I've had only one lover who preferred me to walk around naked while he lit the candles, compared with removing some article of my clothing. Men are really uniform on this one, so throw something over yourself and leave the legs bare.

7. "CATCH ME! I'M A BUTTERFLY." A pointed, raised toe says you are tensed in desire. Take off your shoes, show your cute socks or painted toes, and press down on the ground with the underside of your big toe as though you were wearing toe shoes. The guy sees the arched underside of your foot and gets a little excited. It's up to you whether this is a tease or you're truly interested.

8. "WE ARE A SEXUAL KALEIDOSCOPE." In sex we all like metonymy—part of the body expressing the whole. Try using only your shins and your lips in making love, or suddenly squeeze your ankles against his. Raise your torso away from him while scissoring your legs around his hips. When the sexual dialogue builds this way, the results are very hot.

9. "I THINK OF YOU ALL THE TIME." The brush of a thigh against a man's leg when you're both dressed intoxicates him. So does touching the back of his knee, where the skin is extrasoft.

10. "I'M ALL THE WOMAN YOU'LL EVER NEED." The reason men think they like long legs is that legs lead up to the hips and groin, and a long set of legs suggests a longer trip! In actuality, the petite female who marries the tall lacrosse star has a lot to teach us about making a long trip of his moving up her sexy, expressive legs. The lesson here is to lead a man up from your toes slowly on occasion.

11. "I'M SLEEK AND FOR YOU I'M EASY!" Get in the habit of smoothing a few drops of moisturizer on your legs in anticipation of a hand *en passant* (testing the softness of your skin).

12. "YOU'RE SO HOT I MELT." You don't have to prove how athletic you are. As a woman with legs of above-average muscularity, I made the mistake of almost frightening my big, athletic lover by cinching his body. If you are dainty and feminine this will be meaningless to you, but if you are athletic you may know what I mean. That we may want thighs as strong as the Williams sisters' or as powerful as on a Maillol sculpture doesn't mean we have to use them on a guy. It's a bit of a game to show you're strong but not so strong you could whip him. Men particularly fear being caught in a vulnerable position between potentially disabling female thighs.

13. "I KNOW WHEN YOU THINK SEXY THOUGHTS ABOUT ME." Do you sometimes catch that quicksilver shift from friendly to erotic in your man? You feel the heat on your skin and see the desire in his eyes. You weren't trying to be hot but something ignites. Entice him with a simple movement such as uncrossing and recrossing your legs. The brief moment when the inner thighs are slightly exposed often makes a man's pulse race a bit.

ACCENTUATING YOUR LEGS

There are numerous aspects of the legs that women like and dislike. Here are a few:

- Overall length
- Proportion of legs to length of torso
- Length of knee to ankle versus length of knee to hip (longer lower legs give the illusion of longer legs overall)
- The "two-hole" shape: Ideally, should be able to see daylight above and below the calf muscles when you stand with your legs together
- Shapely ankle: definition, a distinct narrowing from the calf to the anklebone
- Toned, without being overly muscular
- Slim, without looking bony
- Knees: not too knobby, scarred, flabby, or rough-skinned
- Thighs: The big one! A lovely thirty-four-year-old I knew once said that even during hot summer trips she would wear long pants so she wouldn't have to stare at her thighs on the plane or car trip
- Size of thighs: Do they flare out beyond the hips? Do they jiggle? What is the thighs' proportion to bust size? Is the area where thigh becomes butt a definite transition or a flabby, gradual one?
- Appearance and grooming: no hair growth, pretty toenails
- Skin tone, smoothness
- Varicose veins: This is the second big point. One hippie-era woman I know is very earthy but with one vanity, her long, lovely legs, which she has injected with saline solution by a doctor friend every four to six months to diminish the appearance of varicose veins
- Cellulite: Of overriding importance. Today fixable!

All of us are uncomfortable with some aspect of our bodies. Often we look to diet to make an improvement. However,

Great Legs!

vis-à-vis legs, exercise, massage, carriage/movement/walk, cosmetic leg care, foot care, correction of the little flaws by doctors, and choosing outfits that suit us are what enhances our beauty.

We've just set out the ideal. As you look over this list, you'll think, "Yes, that's me" or "No, that isn't me." Now take one nice feature you know you have and think how you can accentuate it. You want to flaunt your inherited traits—it's like the biblical parable of the talents. If your legs are long, show a lot of leg. If they are shapely but heavy, go for a slit in the skirt. If you have nice calves, wear high heels and strappy sandals that draw attention to them. If you tan well or are a woman of color, wear black and white to accentuate that. If you have a "bubble butt" and skinny legs, your figure is perfect for tight jeans.

We are born with a certain "model" of legs. We can make them more beautiful by developing their best traits. Jennifer Lopez is not Charlize Theron. A gymnast is not a high jumper or swimmer. Your legs should look *your* best. Your exercise, your sports, your posture, bathing, cosmetic care, and if you can afford it, massage will give you improved tone, lengthen your body and look, and give you smooth, enviable skin.

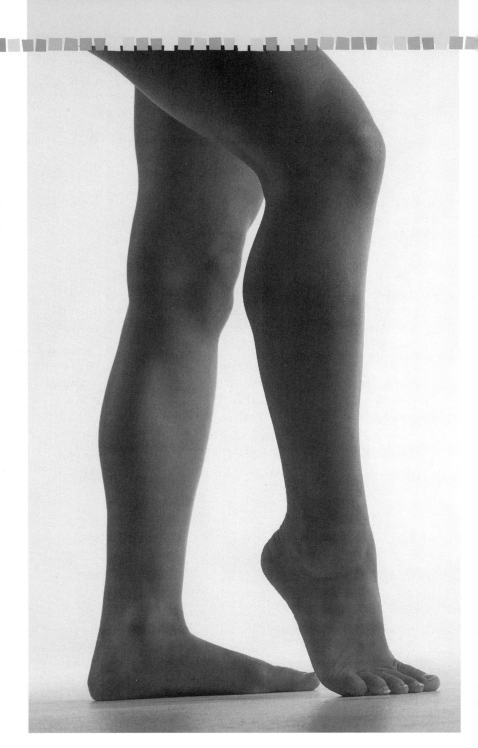

Medical Treatments

Your legs represent a finely tuned walking machine. Your leg and foot bones provide the rigid support needed to keep your body up. Your leg muscles pull your bones in the appropriate direction. Oxygen and nutrients that are essential to power your muscles are delivered to your legs via your blood. This nutrient-rich blood is pumped by the heart and carried in arteries. Arteries are normally smooth and relatively thick and elastic. By avoiding smoking and not eating an excess of foods high in cholesterol, you can help prevent the arteries from becoming stiff and/or narrow (the condition known as atherosclerosis).

After your legs have used the nutrients from the blood, it is returned to the heart and lungs by your veins. Compared with arteries, veins are thinner and less stretchy. One very important difference is that by the time blood has moved through the muscle, skin, or bone and is ready to be returned to the heart, there is very little force left to propel it upward. Also, on the return trip the blood has to fight gravity. Your legs have an ingenious system that uses your calf muscles to pump blood in the veins. There are very thin but effective valves in the veins that prevent the blood from flowing back down the veins when your legs are at rest. If the veins become blocked or the valves break, the pressure in your veins increases and blood can travel the wrong way. This high venous pressure can result in stretched (spider or varicose) veins as well as swelling, heaviness, or achiness in your legs.

Many athletes have prominent superficial veins because they have large muscles and little subcutaneous fat to hide their veins. These veins are usually not abnormal. It's when there's high pressure in the veins that the valves returning the blood to the heart can falter. The following symptoms may indicate a problem with your leg veins:

- Legs aching, feeling heavy, or swelling after prolonged sitting or standing
- Skin itching or weeping at the ankles
- Brownish discoloration of the skin around the ankles and lower calves
- Acute pain and redness, called superficial phlebitis, in the ankles

Women who have had no particular problems with their legs may one day look down and discover they have bad spider veins. Spider veins are smaller than two millimeters. They are within the skin and are primarily a cosmetic concern. Only if they become very extensive will they make your legs feel heavy and achy.

Varicose veins are the stretched or swollen veins that protrude from the surface of the skin. They appear as lumps, bulges, or jagged streaks. If untreated, varicose veins will get more uncomfortable and unsightly. This isn't a life-threatening condition, but it may cause pain and swelling, and certainly does diminish your appearance.

Approximately two-thirds of women end up with at least some small, probably unsightly varicosities in their legs. This condition is most commonly a symptom of old age, obesity, inherited poor valve function, standing for long periods of time, smoking, and even poor diet. Women who are overweight, have frequent pregnancies, take birth control pills, or undergo estrogen and progesterone replacement therapy are also vulnerable to varicosities and spider veins.

Achy, heavy, tired legs caused by spider and varicose veins can be quite effectively treated with lifestyle changes.

You can decide you aren't going to cinch in your waist so circulation is decreased to the lower body. You won't wear tight jeans or panties with killer elastic bands. You won't gain and lose and gain huge amounts of weight. You won't cross your legs or stand for prolonged periods, and you're going to eat so that you're not generally constipated.

Elevate your legs for parts of each day, and switch to low-impact exercise and yoga. If you are required to stand at your job, compression stockings are the answer for work hours. Stockings don't eliminate the varicose veins, but they do prevent swelling and improve the way your legs feel. Compression stockings are also very helpful for pregnant women, who have a higher volume of blood and thus larger veins. "Air cuffs" can also be placed on the feet or legs and inflated several times a minute. You can find these at hospital supply stores. Whichever option you choose, relief is important and can prevent future problems.

ALTERNATIVE TREATMENTS

There are also alternative treatments for the prevention or reduction of spider and varicose veins. Here is a pared-down nondrug protocol I follow. You can purchase many of these supplements at health food stores or online. Take as directed. As with many alternative treatments, none of the healing properties have been proven, and the scientific benefits of the components may not be exactly known. While you should be skeptical of the claims of the companies that sell them, I find the trade association Alchemybotanicals.com useful for picking and choosing what interests me.

COENZYME Q_{10}: This vitamin K–like substance is found naturally in the tissues of all mammals, as is vitamin C. It helps pump energy through us, improves oxygen transport, and regularizes blood pressure. It will aid circulation, thus diminishing the chance of varicose veins appearing.

GRAPE SEED EXTRACT: This substance, an extract of pine bark from France also called Pycnogenol, strengthens connective tissue, especially in the circulatory system. This results in stronger veins, which are less likely to pool blood and thus less likely to appear through the skin.

VITAMIN K: This basic "skin" vitamin prevents bruising and may inhibit spider veins from developing. You can bruise as easily as a peach if you are taking hormone replacement or more baby aspirin, certain supplements, or vitamin K than you need. Doctors have excellent results from K-Derm cream, a dual-purpose topical cream that helps fade spiders on the legs and broken capillaries on the face. Or you might try Vita-K Solution for Spider Veins from the drugstore.

ARNICA: This derivative of vitamin K has been shown to lessen bruising. You can ask your dermatologist for an arnica cream or use Kneipp's cream regularly.

VITAMIN C with bioflavonoids: This vitamin has been shown to keep blood vessels supple.

HORSE CHESTNUT EXTRACT: This is probably the oddest of the supplements listed here, but it is very specific to varicose vein issues. It seems to strengthen capillary walls, protect against vascular damage, and reduce excess fluid in the upper legs and around the ankles.

GOTU KOLA: This herb is also said to improve drainage

in the lymphatic system and prevent redness in the legs. You can find it at several online companies, such as Arrowroot and Nature's Way.

Supplementary vitamins for stronger tone, good circulation, and good health are very worthwhile, according to Dr. Robert Goldman, founder and former president of the American Academy of Sports Medicine. He cautions you to check with your physician before you take them, though, particularly if you are thinking of doing so routinely. The vitamins that Dr. Goldman often recommends as supplements include B_1, or thiamine, for muscle and new tissue; B_2, or riboflavin, and B_6 for skin tone; folic acid, good for circulation, especially in the feet; vitamin C for joints, arteries, and tissue; vitamin E for circulation and skin; and vitamin K for bone mineralization. Ginkgo is good for circulation, aloe vera capsules may improve skin healing, and tinctures of calendula are advisable for scrapes and cuts. (The previous array is a mere sampling.) Be careful with dosages, and note whether the vitamin should be taken at mealtimes. It also makes sense after introducing one supplement to wait a month or so before you add another.

Dr. Mary Bove, a naturopathic family physician and medical herbalist in Brattleboro, Vermont, uses various natural methods to help strengthen the veins. She integrates diet, herbal medicine, nutritional supplements, and hydrotherapy. Besides the bioflavonoids, her approach includes the following recommendations:

- Add walnuts, fresh fish, and a teaspoon of flax oil daily to your diet.
- Take vitamin C with bioflavonoids (500 milligrams daily).
- Take an equal amount of magnesium with your calcium supplement.
- Take 1 teaspoon of blueberry solid fruit extract three times a day.
- Take ginkgo leaf extract (40 milligrams three times a day).

- Put horse chestnut cream on the skin just before bedtime.
- To make yourself feel good, try alternating hot and cold treatments twice a day. Step out of a warm bath into a cool footbath or towel soaked in cold water; or soak one towel hot and one cold and wrap your legs for a minute in each. Afterward splash with witch hazel. The North American Indians discovered that when the leaves and bark of the witch hazel tree are distilled and mixed with alcohol and water, they make a wonderful astringent for burns and inflammations of the skin. This combination also counters itching and tones the skin.

There are currently no FDA-approved medications for the treatment of venous problems. There are, however, many nonapproved medications marketed to patients with vein or leg problems. Most of these creams and pills purport to improve blood flow and increase the tone of the veins. In Europe a product called Daflon, which contains a flavonoid extract, is widely marketed. (Flavonoids are a class of nutrients and vitamins that are one of the active ingredients in grapes and thought to be important for their cardiovascular benefit.) It is very easy to spend hundreds of dollars on creams, lotions, and pills that are widely marketed in publications targeted to women but have no benefits. So beware of these quick-fix treatments.

Dr. Celeste Romig, a dermatologist in Darien, Connecticut, recommends that you go to a dermatologist—the one who treated your child's teenage skin or your poison ivy—and simply ask for a consultation about treatments and prescription-strength products. She says, "It may be you come away with a prescription for a product that will save you money over drugstore brands because it is more effective."

Dr. Nicholas Perricone is a research dermatologist and award-winning inventor who has done three PBS specials and has dozens of U.S. and international patents on antioxidants and anti-inflammatory medicines to counter the effects of aging. Under his pharmaceutical label he has a thigh toner and body cream with some of the same antiaging ingredients as face products. Dr. Perricone's Anti-Spider Veins is a blend of alpha lipoic acids designed to diminish the appearance of spider veins while toning and firming the skin. If you have a spider problem but eschew surgery, try Dr. Perricone's cream for sixty days.

From a small pharmaceutical outfit comes the Nu Visage line, with the Complete Leg and Vein Therapy Regimen, which has an oral supplement to strengthen the veins internally and a restorative leg cream. The products, made with a compound derived from grape seed and pine bark imported from France, rebuild and protect collagen in the skin and repair another key enzyme, elastin, in both the skin and connective tissues. Nu Visage makes no claims that their products reverse vein damage, but they do reverse the sluggishness in aging legs.

If your spider veins are no more than the width of a thin piece of yarn, the best remedy is to try the least costly and troublesome solution, then if necessary, move up the scale. If you use Dr. Perricone's product for a few months, you may well find that your spiders are no more noticeable than a string in the pitch dark.

SURGICAL TREATMENTS

Spider veins can be surgically treated by two methods, sclerotherapy or laser therapy. You should be sure the doctor you consult is experienced in both these options.

Sclerotherapy uses injections of a salt solution (saline) or a soaplike solution (sodium tetradecyl sulfate, SDS). Polidoconal, perhaps the most effective and safest agent, is not at present approved by the FDA. The injections are done, using a very small needle, directly into the spider veins. Since the solution spreads, a single injection can often treat several inches of veins. The solution works by irritating the inner lining of the vein, causing it to close down. Once the vein is scarred closed, it disappears and blood is rerouted through tributary veins.

This treatment causes relatively minor discomfort and is quite effective. You can typically expect about two-thirds of the veins treated at any one session to be effectively eliminated. Limited spider veins can be treated in one session, but extensive spiders may require several sessions. If the solution leaks from the damaged vein, you may experience brown spots or small ulcers on the skin. These are almost always dime-size or smaller and will disappear with simple bandaging or ointment.

Laser therapy is the second medical option for treating spider veins. A laser is flashed through the skin like a flashlight. The light is filtered to a wavelength that makes the blood (hemoglobin) vibrate and thus heat up. The heated blood damages the vein and causes it to close. However, unlike sclerotherapy solutions, the laser energy does not spread; spiders must be lasered along their entire length.

Each laser pulse covers about two millimeters and causes mild discomfort, similar to being struck with a rubber band. The discomfort can be alleviated by cooling the skin. In addition, the laser treatment can cause inflammation that leaves red streaks over the veins, but it usually fades in days to weeks. Bruising may also occur, and skin may lighten. Lightening of the skin (hypopigmentation) is primarily an issue for dark-complexioned women; usually the skin recovers in weeks to months, but it may not return completely to normal.

After sclero or laser treatments, it's recommended that you keep your legs moisturized and wrapped for a few days. Walking is okay, but no vigorous activity, like running or biking, is recommended for two weeks. Also, sun exposure should be limited.

Sclerotherapy is preferable for women with veins large enough to reliably inject greater than a one-millimeter area.

Great Legs!

This treatment is faster, less painful, and more effective. Smaller veins are better treated with a laser except in dark-skinned women.

For varicose veins, relatively minor surgery or nonsurgical treatments can often alleviate the problem. The initial evaluation is best carried out by a vascular surgeon familiar with all stages and types of venous disease. Once an acute condition is ruled out, what is called for is either injection with a medication that shrinks the veins down to size or surgical stripping. These procedures have short recovery periods and are almost pain-free.

The new treatment options can be an embarrassment of riches unless you have the judgment of an experienced specialist. To get your teenage legs back, you should go to a surgeon who treats similar cases day in and day out.

LATEST TECHNIQUES

Two techniques that have emerged, which are a godsend for varicose veins, are EndoVenous Laser Treatment and radio frequency ablation. The radio frequency procedure is trademarked Closure. The difference between these methods is the type of energy delivery. A laser heats the blood and indirectly heats the vein. Radio frequency generates heat at the tips of small probes that actually touch the vein walls. Both treatments cause vein wall injury and contraction, and eliminate blood flow so the varicose veins disappear. These procedures are done only in large veins. However, if the main vein is treated, there is typically decreased pressure in *all* the varicose veins lower in the leg.

Dr. Romig tells us that "lasers work wonders on leg veins. There are several wavelengths we can use, depending on the color and diameter of the veins. Three or four treatments are required, with minimal bruising as the only side effect. They can even be safely performed during pregnancy!"

Dr. Romig explains, "The lasers we use in dermatology act

from the *outside* of the veins and deliver energy to cauterize or destroy them. Endovascular lasers act from the *inside* of the veins and are used for treating severe varicose veins in a hospital setting."

Radiofrequency is another way of delivering energy to a vein or lesion in order to change or destroy it. Lasers use light energy as opposed to radiofrequency or sound wave. The end result is the same, just a different source of energy. Wavelengths of light that are absorbed by the red pigment are used to destroy blood vessels in the skin. Wavelengths of light that are absorbed by brown pigments are used to remove freckles and age spots. Wavelengths of light that are absorbed by green or blue are used for tattoo removal.

When catheter ablation was performed, more than one-half of the patients noticed improvement and underwent no further treatments. For this process the catheter is placed into the vein through a needle and guided by ultrasound. Local anesthesia is used at the puncture site. The catheter is inserted near the knee and typically guided to a position in the groin. Additional local anesthesia and saline are injected through the skin to surround the vein in the area to be treated. This compresses the vein and also absorbs the heat so nearby nerves and skin are not injured. The catheter is then drawn back slowly (ten to twenty minutes) while the vein is heated.

After any of these techniques, you can expect to have your legs wrapped in elastic wraps for a day or two. You may have some stiffness and soreness, but most patients state that the pain is much less than they expected.

Both of these procedures are 90 percent effective in the short term. No long-term data are available yet, but the procedures seem durable for at least two to three years. Charges for these procedures vary widely. Most insurance carriers now cover radio-frequency ablation for symptomatic varicose veins; however, many do not cover the laser option.

If you are going to undergo these high-tech treatments, it's crucial to put your legs in the right hands. Vascular programs at hospitals like Tufts–New England Medical Center in Boston offer the convenience of one facility for treating all leg concerns.

There is simply no reason to be discouraged by those protruding lines on your legs, as the options for their safe removal are both plentiful and accessible. The vein system has a lot of redundancy, and if the bad veins are eliminated, the remaining good veins function even better. Therefore, if bad veins are removed or closed, circulation in the legs actually improves.

I simply recommend that you become as educated as possible about your vein problem so you can address it in the most appropriate manner. Here are five questions to ask whatever the procedure:

• What is the doctor's experience in this specific treatment?
• What diagnostics are used and why?
• What about recovery time?
• Could the condition recur?
• What is the cost?

Be sure if you consult a physician that he or she presents you with alternatives. There is no single perfect solution for spiders and varicose veins, but there are therapies that will answer your needs.

EXTREME LEG BEAUTY

Cosmetic surgery is a miracle at best, a curse at worst. If you are seriously unhappy with your thighs or other aspects of your legs, you'll want to find a cosmetic surgeon who is greatly involved in body contouring, with outstanding artistic talent and superb medical and surgical skills. Ask for referrals. Then ask to see some "before and after" pictures. The doctor will have these untouched photos, which do not lie. I have looked at many doctors' work, and most of the time I believe the person looked better before she went under the knife. That's a shame but a fact, so beware.

For this book I went to the most august beauty magician I could find, Dr. Joseph Pober, who is one of Park Avenue's top cosmetic surgeons. When I saw the before and after shots in Dr. Pober's book, I was amazed. He makes ordinary women into extraordinary beauties. I think "Pygmalion!" Then, as he educates me, I realize his worldwide success comes from addressing beauty on many planes and keeping his specialty, surgery, in reserve for when it's truly called for.

Among many distinguished medical peers, Dr. Pober is undoubtedly the Leonardo da Vinci. He is a prizewinning painter of portraits of women as well as trained to give women the faces and bodies they desire (and can afford). Movie stars and celebrities beat a path to his door for his low-invasive techniques, some of which he has innovated, but also for his aesthetics of creating a natural look.

Thanks to the doctor's graciousness, I'm taking you virtually into his consulting room for the surprising skinny on what to do and not to do from the point of view of a master of the highest tech contouring of our legs, knees, and thighs.

DR. POBER SPEAKS ON
THE BEAUTY LEG SCENE

Leg beauty has three components in medical terms: the bone structure, which predetermines your general shape; the musculature, which can be developed substantially by various exercise routines; and a layer of fat. So many women are so active with their exercise that I find it sometimes works against them, simply because it makes them too muscular.

The style today is long, slim legs, yet the ways available to obtain them are often limited by the women themselves. Women can restrict the changes we doctors offer them. For instance, if you do too much quad work, you extend your knees too frequently and start building up a muscle that rides atop your leg. Demi Moore had a wrinkle on top of her knee that was probably a result of exercising too much. If you overexercise your quads, I recommend you incorporate a variety of exercises that will start reducing those muscles and also those little creases, which in a male may be appealing but in a female become lines.

The other concern from exercising is that you may develop enormous thighs or calves. A significant proportion of women end up with stocky, short, knobby legs. Exercise can help reconfigure your legs. To have pretty, well-proportioned legs, the best kind of exercise I recommend is zero resistance, or almost no resistance, as in bicycle riding. Simply getting on a bicycle and moving your legs will give you attractive looking gams. If your thighs or calves are thundering, your best tactic of all is to go dancing. Ballroom dancing or jazz dancing will give you longer, leaner legs.

Running and jogging are trickier. There is too much pounding, especially on pavement or a hard surface, without proper cushioning for your foot. If you are jogging you are causing the skin on your thighs to go up and down. The same thing is happening all over your body. Your knees start to look saggy. When patients come to me for leg reshaping, I look first at their exercise routine. So many women come in saying, "I have a trainer. We're doing squats. We're doing heavy lifting. I'm able to move a hundred pounds with my legs and I only weigh a hundred pounds." I say, "No wonder you look so terrible! Building your muscles to a high degree made your legs tight as a drum, but you're bulky. If you desire long, thin legs, you must change your routine. The weight you have noticed is not fat but muscle mass, which cannot be surgically removed."

Legs, though, from a physical point of view, are forgiving. If you have gained bulk, I recommend a cooling-down period of three to six months, when you do zero-resistance workouts. Dancing, walking, and fast running are okay, but jogging is out. Cycling is out; try the indoor bikes with zero resistance. I like a patient to try adjusting her exercise before she comes to me. After she is left with only fat, muscle, and the basic bone structure, we can perform liposuction or body changes to achieve the look she wants.

The standard of beauty that patients want is based on the standard of our culture: a rounded look and not a great deal of definition. Notice that swimmers, whose sport has some but not very high resistance, have beautiful legs. Volleyball and tennis shape legs nicely for the same reason, lots of movement, low resistance. By contrast, if you run marathons, you will have tubular legs when young and by your thirties some sagging muscles, which will be a problem in your fifties.

Your leg shape is determined by structure, posture, and walk. How you walk and move is critical. If you move your legs in a way that is appealing to you, they will look nicer. I recommend you exercise in front of a mirror. If you are doing an exercise that looks as though you're straining, or has you contorted or looking unattractive, the result for your legs will be awkward. Seeing that you look nice while you exercise is actually critical.

DR. POBER EXPLAINS SPECIFIC
CONDITIONS AND HIS RECOMMENDATIONS

The newest and hottest techniques rely on minimally invasive microsurgery. These leave either no scar or a "pinhole" scar. The access points are at crease lines, so they can be camouflaged. We can now modify delicate features on the face with techniques that lend themselves very nicely to larger structures, like the legs. We can fine-tune by the addition and removal of fat. Sometimes fat can be enhancing.

Toxic deposits of cellulite accumulate in the fatty tissues around the waist, hips, buttocks, upper arms, and legs. When you feel a bit lumpy, first realize that taking off a few pounds may reduce the obvious. However, it's rigorous self-massage, lymphatic therapy by a certified specialist, or liposuction that really gets rid of fatty tissue. If, like me, you eat refined sugar, drink tea, coffee, carbonated beverages, and alcohol, you are a candidate for cellulite. If you eat raw vegetables and fruit each day, and drink a lot of water, you help the lymphatic system do its job and may avert cellulite.

Self-massage is great for cellulite reduction. Not trained in massage? Just remember your objectives: to stimulate sluggish circulation and flush water out from your system. When you rub in your massage cream or essential oil blend, use long strokes up from the knee. When your lubrication has penetrated, use more brisk and firm strokes, such as hacking (which leads with the heels of your hands), cupping (the noisy one that feels softer than it sounds), and pummeling with the base of your fists. If you are sincere about wanting to say good-bye to cellulite, you'll find the moments in your day for the self-massage. Do it when you're stuck in traffic or at a long stoplight. Three minutes is plenty; frequency is the key.

In conclusion, Dr. Pober does not object to patients using my favorite cellulite product, Dr. Perricone's Body Toning Lotion (SP15 with NTP complex with DMAE), available at fancy department stores or online. I also suggest rose geranium essential oil for its slight diuretic property. Put 4 drops in the juice of 2 fresh lemons and rub some over your knees for the mild bleaching effect. There are also high-end cosmetics you can try. Bliss has a section in their catalog of "Girth Control" products that includes an anti-cellulite mud mask and a cream with an "exclusive bromo-iodine cocktail created from the mineralized salt waters surrounding the celebrated Salsomaggiore Spa." Their Elysse Rollercell also features motorized rollers, deep heat, and vibration massage.

MESOTHERAPY

Slimming, toning, and smoothing will make most of us happy about our legs. However, if cellulite really causes you duress, I suggest a treatment that has been around for fifty years in Europe and is gaining credence here, mesotherapy. Dr. Lionel Bissoon, the leading expert in the United States, despite his relative youth, has trained the first generation of mesotherapists. He also pioneered a form of mesotherapy called Stringcision, a minimally invasive procedure to eliminate dimples that appear on the buttocks and thighs as a result of cellulite.

Through a series of ten to fifteen treatments, women see a permanent reduction in the poochy skin. Explains Dr. Bissoon, "Most doctors couldn't care less about cellulite. They tell women to just live with it. Mesotherapy is the only medical treatment for cellulite. Liposuction has merits but doesn't work for cellulite—as any proper cosmetic surgeon will tell you. The mechanical massages don't work either."

What mesotherapy does is remedy the unsightly "dented" area by vitalizing it. Pharmaceutical and homeopathic medications and nutrients including minerals, vitamins, and amino acids are injected into the problem area. The principle is that decreased estrogen results in poor circulation as well as damaged collagen and connective tissue, followed by fat cells herniating through the connective tissue, thus producing cellulite. The "cocktail" of mesotherapy repairs the damaged fine mesh that lets fat cells through, increasing circulation and shrinking fat cells.

Dr. Bissoon points out that women who are active outdoors do not have cellulite. He believes that it comes from three negatives: living a sedentary live, eating foods with many additives, and wearing underwear that has elastic. "Tight jeans aren't nearly as bad," he advises. "The panties with elastic bands produce localized compression and cause dimples in the buttocks."

The three preventions Dr. Bissoon suggests are to exercise for shorter periods but twice a day, emphasize natural foods in your diet, and check for those telltale red lines when you undress. If your panty elastic is constricting your buttocks or thighs, jettison the underwear! (Information about Dr. Bissoon and his book *The Cellulite Cure* can be found at www.mesotherapy.com.)

From high-end cosmetics companies come certain products that seriously claim to reduce cellulite. Unfortunately, no scientific study proves any of these products to be efficacious at the present time. These products are not to be dabbled in; if you are going to experiment, you have to use them religiously as the purveyors recommend. Products such as Biotherm's Celluli-Choc often contain caffeine to dilate the blood vessels and increase circulation. Other products have algae for the high silicone content, which detoxifies and makes the body supple. Still others may contain ingredients like wheat protein to tighten the skin, paraffin to hydrate (Clinique's Firming Body Smoother is based on water therapy), and proprietary elements that stimulate enzymes to break down fat. For example, Aromaflora's Tighten and Tone Treatment Gel has sea minerals and marine extracts, and Algotherm's Firming and Slimming Gel is also made from sea-derived concentrates such as Algo-Silicon, seaweed extract, and spirulina algae.

What will a spa do for you? Let's look at what the Sea Change Healing Center in New York has to offer for an anti-cellulite routine:

SEA CHANGE ANTI-CELLULITE WELLNESS PACKAGE

Help is here for the prevention and removal of cellulite—the buildup of toxins in the system manifested in old fat cell clusters, nasty orange peel skin, and cottage cheese thighs. This collaborative wellness program assists in the prevention and elimination of cellulite with a three-step program including a diet detox, Chinese medicine, and massage therapy.

PART 1: 3-week detox program
PART 2: 6 sessions of Chinese medicine
PART 3: 6 sessions of 1-hour lymphatic massage

PART 1: DETOX

To ward off cellulite you must rid the system of toxins and toxic buildup, and make sure that no further toxins build up in your system and that wastes are being eliminated properly. Detoxifying the body with a nutritional fast is vital in jump-starting the system into wellness. A naturopathic physician supervises the 3-week detox program.

PART 2: CHINESE MEDICINE

This portion of the program includes the removal of cellulite with a combination of an ancient Chinese technique called cupping and a special all-natural herbal fat-burning cream. A vacuum cupping method utilizes a plastic jar attached to a handheld pump. Once a partial vacuum is created in a jar, it is applied to the skin and the underlying tissues are drawn up. Then the cup is slid on target areas to create negative pressure to break down the fatty deposit. The suction also helps to speed up the absorption of cream by increasing the blood circulation. Cupping is a unique therapeutic modality within Chinese medicine to heal, rather than simply relax the body and relieve tension. Acupuncture needles may be used for some patients. For maximized achievement, 6 treatment sessions (1 session a week for 6 weeks) are recommended along with a wellness lifestyle program. Each treatment lasts about 30 minutes.

PART 3: MASSAGE

The best type of massage for cellulite is a Sea Change Lymphatic Drainage Massage. This treatment includes gentle, rhythmic pumping movements and massage designed to stimulate the lymph system. Utilizing therapeutic drainage techniques, tissue is gently pumped and cleansed of wastes and toxins, breaking down fat stored and lessening fat deposits. This massage improves the flow of lymph and enhances healing and circulation. Your therapist also massages specific reflexology points on your hands and feet to accelerate lymph drainage. This massage is excellent for reducing pain and swelling, fluid retention, chronic inflammation, sinus conditions, headaches, and sprains. Our special blend of tangerine and grapefruit essential oils is designed to help digest fat cells, which is important in breaking down cellulite. Grapefruit essential oil increases fat-dissolving actions in areas of fat rolls, puckers, and dimples. Since cellulite is slow to dissolve, we suggest clients commit to having 1 massage per week during a 6-week period, beginning the first week of the detox program.

LIPOSUCTION

Liposuction, when done right, is medical artistry. This procedure used to be major surgery but now associated morbidity and complications are almost nonexistent. Vision correction used to be a "miracle" operation; now there are doctors vying for our business on the radio. Lasering off hair used to be in doctors' hands only. Now there are laser parlors. Botox is moving down the echelons too. And now liposuction is being done on our thighs, calves, and the backs of knees with only local anesthesia. Cosmetic surgeons can shape thighs. This is sometimes called lipocontouring, to emphasize the three-dimensionality of the approach.

Liposuction is for women who have gone as far as they can with diet and exercise, and still have unattractive fat on their legs. All cosmetic surgeons do liposuction routinely, but you want a doctor experienced in aesthetic subtle alterations. The goal is lovely contours, not the etching of unnatural depressions. Make sure you ask to see photographs of the surgeon's results. Also, your legs should be examined and analyzed as whole three-dimensional structures. The doctor should consider the proportions (thighs thicker than knees, knees a little thinner than calves, calves a little larger than ankles, and so forth). You want to end up with a slow, natural transition in the contour of the buttocks to upper thighs, and an overall more aesthetically pleasing silhouette. The cosmetic surgeon Dr. Joseph Pober explains in his new textbook that the surgeon will view the thigh as a "rectangle . . . to be sculpted or lipocarved to create a pleasing anatomical shape."

Small changes require the most skilled surgeon. Dr. Pober explains: "You're so close to what you want to be. It's not just a matter of debulking with standard liposuction, but getting aesthetically pleasing results. These techniques are never for people who are just out of shape and are trying to get into shape. Lipocontouring is for areas of fat that are resistant to diet and exercise, and for people who've worked very hard but want more."

There are two things that medical technology will never be able to do for our legs. The first is establish aesthetic standards. Those combine nature and fashion. The second is create another you, with your unique bone structure and musculature. Whatever leg solutions you choose, the idea is to enhance not erase.

Cellulite seems to arise in women who have undergone weight fluctuations, not necessarily extreme changes but multiple fluctuations. The various therapies work to draw out the fat so it flushes away. You will see that this condition is treatable not curable.

Surgery for cellulite yields a visible change. Because it's done through a pinhole, there is no scarring. Basically the surgery breaks up the structure. It also removes excess fat in the desired compartments.

Legs are so quick to respond to exercise, massage, and pampering. Fluid retention is the major reason cellulite shows, so you can make it look better with stimulation and flushing it out. One technique, called Endermologie, is popular with doctors. It uses rollers and suction to massage cellulite areas. It's not a cure but a maintenance program for legs, recommended for ages twenty to sixty. You go twice a week for a month, then once a month. Afterward it's recommended you drink more than the usual amount of fluids through the day. This treatment can bring down the fatty deposits of the body, especially on the arms, legs, and thighs. Endermologie, declares Dr. Ron Shelton, of the New York Aesthetic Center, actually shrinks that volume. "This is for the scalpel- and anesthesia-shy. It feels more natural and gives improvement in most patients. You may get more results than you expect."

When it comes down to it, liposuction is for those of us whose legs require results that regular exercise and healthy eating cannot provide. Given the current level of artistry and competition among plastic surgeons, you can be sure that there is a doctor capable of performing the procedure you require.

WARTS

A wart is caused by a virus in the skin. Fortunately, warts can be treated with medication. Always start with an over-the-counter method. After two months if it's not gone, Dr. Romig says to see your dermatologist. In her opinion you should not have the CO_2 treatment sometimes used to remove warts, because it can scar. Freezing is the treatment often favored by dermatologists because it is the least likely to leave a scar. The process uses a liquid nitrogen formula and is a painless office procedure. Sometimes the dermatologist will also prescribe a topical cream.

Dermatologists also report using pulsed dye laser treatment, particularly for multiple warts. It involves no needles or bleeding. However, several sessions are usually needed, two to four weeks apart. For the laser beam to penetrate elevated warts that are covered with thick calluses or deep plantar warts on the bottoms of the feet, the growths must first be pared down with a scalpel. There is a small risk of scarring with this option.

Many insurance companies do not reimburse patients for pulsed dye laser treatment unless conventional therapies fail. However, for some patients, it may be worth the out-of-pocket expense for a better cosmetic result. To prevent warts, I recommend if you wear shorts when you work out at a gym to use an antiseptic body wash on your knees and any portion of the leg that may have contacted a bench or mat. Rubber sandals or flip-flops are a must to wear when showering at the gym to prevent warts from forming on your feet. I also believe you can speed up the healing of warts by using supplements like vitamins E and K.

STRETCH MARKS

Stretch marks occur when collagen and elastin fibers in the dermis, or inner layer of the skin, are torn. As you gain weight or exercise intensely, the skin stretches and its elastic fibers rupture. Appearing first as bands of wrinkled skin, they are pink, red, or purple streaks that later become silvery white. Since the tendency to get them is at least partly heredity, there is no way to prevent stretch marks 100 percent.

Stretch marks are typically caused by pregnancy, adolescent growth spurts, weight lifting, or rapid weight gain. Steroids and estrogen also seem to play a role in their development. Stretch marks on the abdomen are usually tokens of having borne a child but are also caused by significant weight gain and loss. However, on the legs stretch marks can form as the results of intense workouts, such as bodybuilding. Women in their late teens and twenties can have stretch marks on their legs, hips, and buttocks that eventually fade later. So there's no cause to seek aggressive treatment right away. But if they do not fade, stretch marks can be healed by laser treatment. Unfortunately, the effect may not be permanent. Many women may have to have the treatment repeated a few years later if they want to stay stretch mark free.

Another treatment that gets approbation from dermatological studies is the topical application of a high-strength vitamin C solution.

In addition to the vascular-specific lasers, the high-energy, rapidly pulsed resurfacing lasers are sometimes helpful in improving the appearance of stretch marks. (Ask the dermatologist about carbon dioxide or erbium:YAG lasers.) The medical literature suggests that stretch marks may also diminish with the daily application of Retin-A or alpha hydroxy acids; hence these agents, applied at home, are often used in conjunction with laser treatment.

Dr. Ron Shelton, of the New York Aesthetic Center, says

there is an optimal time to make stretch marks vanish with laser. Once they lose their redness, it's too late. After pregnancy, the red marks may last a few months or a year or more. You don't want to be lasered while you are nursing, plus they may go away by themselves. Take a look at six months; it might be the time to laser them to oblivion.

Some topical products to treat stretch marks include Mei camellia seed oil (victani.com) and Streiveichten. Do you like the exotic ingredients as much as I do? According to victani.com, "The Mei camellia seed oil is found in the winter wild flowers of China and Japan. This natural plant oil contains antioxidants to help revitalize the skin. Camellia flowers ripen their luscious seed for a year producing spectacular colors of white, pink, and red. This seed or "fruit" of the camellia is harvested and cold pressed to produce pure, natural camellia seed oil."

A very comely member of my family remarried at age thirty-seven and told her husband, "No children, no stretch marks, I decline the whole package!" I thought, "She married a prosperous man. He adores her and she never has to work again. He'll love his beautiful wife's stretch marks, why care?"

Now I have a different perspective. My friend Susan was the director of public relations PR for a high-end cosmetics company when she married in her late twenties. Each of two pregnancies she gained a whopping sixty-five pounds. Because she massaged cocoa butter into her belly daily, she didn't get a single stretch mark . . . there. However, you can get them *anywhere*. "Had I taken precautions!" she sighs, admitting the stretch marks on her rear and breasts make her lower the lights during sex today. I feel it's fair to say no woman wants to find herself with stretch marks. So use the cocoa butter, don't tan them into greater visibility, and if it is an important issue to you, discuss the alternatives for removing stretch marks with your dermatologist.

KNEES

We tend to think about the health of our knees only when they hurt. Do you look down and feel like the Tin Man—where's the oil can? I expected that a top orthopedic surgeon would give me a ton of cautionary advice about knees, but instead I hear revolutionary thoughts.

Dr. Kevin Plancher is a young orthopedic knee surgeon in New York, trained at Zulu University, who treks every summer to the Arctic Circle on his knees. He gives us the following advice:

Today women's concerns about their knees are *athletic*—it's exciting! Like any body part, the knees need to warm up. You need the blood to flow through the knees to perform at a peak level.

For whatever reason (it may be hormonal, diabetic, or hereditary), some of us get thick, callused skin on our knees. Many women put up with rough knees, not realizing they are easily treated. There is a group of medications called keratolytics that dissolve the layers of skin that have gotten "gluey." There are AHA (glycolic) products, urea products like Carmol or Vanamide, and salicylic acid creams. Some of the same products can work on roughened ankles. Since the skin is layered, and it takes about thirty days to penetrate a layer, it takes about three months to see any results.

Even if you cross train and warm up, you may have aching knees at some point. You'll let up on some activities naturally, but if the pain kicks in, coenzyme DD_4 can be injected into the knee. It's not just analgesic but good for your health, because it keeps the knee functioning smoothly. If your knee aches, it could also be from torn ligaments, stress from too much weight (that you carry on your own), or mechanical problems like one leg being shorter or an infinitesimal misalignment of the knee.

As soon as you feel pain, ice. Keep ice packs in the freezer.

HOW DO
Your Legs
LIKE YOU TO SIT?

There is a chair design so magnificent for your gams that every office worker should consider using it for part of every day. The kneeling chair was designed in the early 1980s by an ergonomic specialist but really gained notice in the late nineties. In 1998 Jobri gained the manufacturing rights from one of the earliest developers. They are now the largest manufacturer of kneeling chairs in the United States. Their kneeling chair is the most reasonably priced and elegantly designed. It looks neat with you on it or when tucked under your desk. You may want to kick off your shoes for total comfort when perching happily on your kneeling chair. The chairs come in wood with upholstery pads, but you can get other looks too. They come as kits and take fifteen minutes to assemble; tools are included. For more information, go to www.jobri.com.

If you are not home, find a store with frozen vegetables and use a bag of frozen peas.

Ice twice a day—15 minutes each time, 5 on, 5 off, 5 on again. The next day, use a hot compress or heating pad. Take ibuprofen for the swelling, and to soothe and relax the muscles.

If more aggressive treatment seems required, anti-inflammatory medications are recourses. When a knee is painful, instead of the usual painkillers, you can get an injection of hyaluronate. This is a thick fluid that your body manufactures. It is also extracted from roosters' combs. Originally used to treat horses after they raced, hyaluronate helps lubricate the joint.

A ginger extract supplement also helps achy knees. The active ingredient, gingerol, reduces pain and increases function. My son takes ginger in the spring, knowing he'll be more active then in sports.

Other preventative supplements are glucosamine and chondroitin. Take up to 1500 milligrams a day for a month to six weeks. It's believed that these not only halt the decrease in cartilage but also increase cartilage in the joints.

While most of us do ignore our knees until we can barely stand, with the information in this section you can begin a preemptive attack on knee pain. We can only hope that by following this advice closely we will never have to deal with the knee problems associated with middle age or intensive exercise.

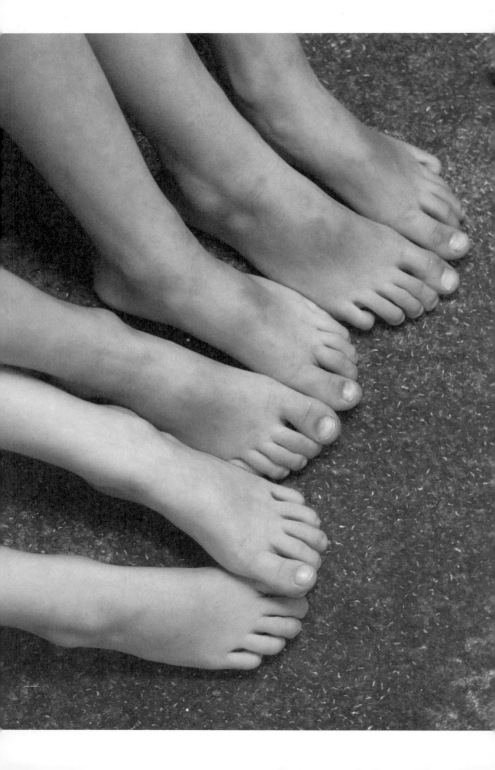

PART II

Feet

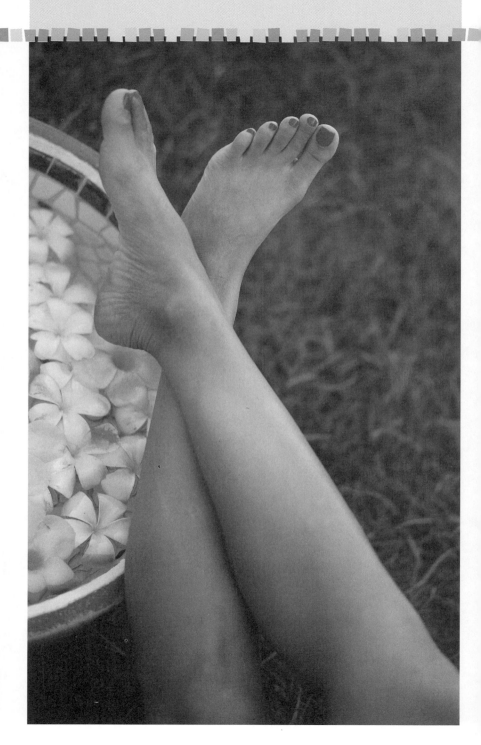

Home Foot Treatments

I BELIEVE IT is important that women know how to treat themselves right, without having to rely on spa and doctor visits. So I have compiled a comprehensive review of the best spa-grade ingredients and techniques for your feet. Applied on a regular basis, these tips can substitute for those expensive spa visits.

Shea butter is basic to your foot beauty routine. It can now be found in many cosmetics lines. It's soft, not oily, and effective but not greasy. This butter glides on. You can apply it at night and it feels like a coating, yet when you wake up it doesn't feel oily. Your feet will be so happy if you put on shea butter at night, sometimes even with booties.

Herbal booties intended to be worn to bed are also called foot mittens. Some foot mittens have herbs sewn into one layer; they're kind of like sacheted drawer papers. There are electric versions that are nice for perpetually cold feet, but be careful you don't burn your feet if you like these little toasters. Since bacteria thrive on warmth, it's obviously necessary to take extra care washing and drying before you give your feet a warm butter treat. Whichever type of treatment you choose, your feet will surely thank you.

If you neglect everything you are about to learn and your feet get cracks like the parting of the Red Sea, opt for a medical solution. Mupirocin is a prescription antibacterial that promotes truly fast healing and is not greasy. Dr. Celeste Romig recommends applying Mupirocin before bedtime and then putting on socks to increase the absorption.

You can't be a mover and a shaker when your feet ache. Try Tipton Charles Bath & Massage Oil in Ocean, Grapefruit, or Mandarin-Guava. Take care of your soles with a stellar antiseptic formula like Carmol, which acts against roughness and moisturizes. Look for products containing urea. Enrich with aloe, safflower oil, seaweed, sage leaf, horse chestnut, vitamins, eucalyptus, and menthol to soften hard skin and fight athlete's foot.

SUPPLEMENTS

You can get supplements designed to keep your eyes bright and nourish your hair, but there is no formula to magically revamp your feet. The usual attention to enough water, fruits, and vegetables in your diet suffices. Here are a few recommendations for specific foot matters.

ARNICA Homeopaths treat what ails you with what ails you. If you have any medical procedures done, ask your doctor if you can take arnica right beforehand orally or as a lotion or cream. The idea is the arnica bruises infinitesimally, which alerts your body to send healing. Arnica is promoted for its antiseptic and soothing qualities.

TEA TREE OIL This antiseptic oil has been mentioned in conjunction with preventing bacterial infection. Tea tree oil in a lotion will also keep the bugs away. It is scientifically proven to reduce the volume of allergic inflammation and anecdotally claimed to help heal cuts or scars.

VITAMIN E If I or one of my children have a cut, burn, or scar, I open a vitamin E capsule and apply it directly to the affected spot. Many plastic surgeons prescribe vitamin E to accelerate healing of the skin. However, the American College of Dermatologists has issued a statement that vitamin E has no known usefulness medically or cosmetically and notes that some people can be allergic to it when directly applied to the skin.

Foot soaks are an additional treat for tired feet. Vary your soak with the season and your whim. Here is the basic mixture concocted by my friend Roberta Boyle at Green Valley Aromatherapy Ltd. This Canadian company is a very reliable source for massage oils and basic skin care. They have body care formulas that you can personalize and perfume as you choose.

FOOT SOAK RECIPE

1 1/2 cups Epsom salts (available at any pharmacy)

3 drops of any of the following oils:

- Lavender (to relax)
- Peppermint (to energize)
- Tea tree (to treat foot fungus or odor problems)

Add the oil to a footbath filled with comfortably warm or hot water. Add the salts and dissolve. Soak your feet until the water becomes cool.

A lot of people are on the brink of fungal infections and don't even know it. If you think you may have one, mix tea tree oil, which is stimulating and invigorating, into a light and breathable foot cream. I like Caswell-Massey's, or Get Fresh's Foot Rescue. Disinfect as you stimulate and invigorate your feet.

PEDICURE

If you had the time and money, you'd probably have a professional pedicure every Friday at four. A weekly pedicure is your feet's desire, so sometimes go to a nail salon, sometimes do it yourself. There are ways to make the care and decoration of your feet both entertaining and relaxing. Transport a basin of warm water to a cozy chair or couch and situate yourself. While you're soaking your feet, read a trashy magazine or a poetry book. Call a friend and chat, or put cucumber slices or pads on your eyes while your feet indulge in the warm water. Your feet will get pretty, and you'll feel brand-new. This could be one of your favorite new routines.

A note on creams and oils: You'll have to customize according to what pampers the nails of your tootsies best. These days a cream is not just a cream when it comes to nails. The toenail is relatively thick—otherwise it would break. When you use an oil it covers the moisture that is in the nails already, as well as smoothes the nail's surface and makes the cuticles supple. Creams, on the other hand, basically moisturize. They may be blended with AHA that exfoliates and strengthens or revitalizes the outer layer, and they sometimes contain "cuticle oil" as well. Additionally, a cream may have sunscreen.

Each nail cream is *tailored:* Read the label and make your judgment call. What do *you* want? Your girlfriend may want the UV protection because she is going on a cruise, whereas you may have good skin texture on your feet and prefer just a nongreasy, light oil that you apply with a cotton swab when your feet are still moist from bathing time. It's fun to personalize all the elements of your pedicure and foot-care regimen from heel to toe!

FOR A PEDICURE YOU WILL NEED
• A dish with a teaspoon each of tea tree oil and vegetable or mineral oil

- A rectangular washbasin—a dish basin is fine; a metal one from a pharmacy is even better, since metal holds heat.
- Bath salts or bath soak
- Cotton balls
- Nail polish remover (if you're wearing old polish)
- Big emery board (not metal) or nail clippers
- Towel
- Cuticle oil
- Cuticle stick
- Cuticle cream
- Pumice stone
- Moisturizer
- Two pieces of facial tissue
- Colored polish
- A clear top coat polish
- Blow dryer (optional)

It makes sense to keep these items in the basin for quick retrieval. Otherwise you'll spend as long collecting stuff as giving yourself the pedicure.

STEP 1

Wash your feet and apply the oil mixture between your toes. This step disinfects your feet. Fill the basin halfway with warm water and bath salts or soak and carry it to your designated spot. Use the cotton balls and nail polish remover to remove any old polish. Then file your nails with the emery board. Do this straight across each nail, not curving down at the sides. If you do this less often than once a week, you'll need to clip the nails instead.

STEP 2

Soak.

STEP 3

Remove one foot and dry with your towel. Apply cuticle oil to the cuticle area along the bottom of each toenail to smooth and remove any flakiness from the nails. Push back the cuticles gently with a cuticle stick. If doing this hurts, wrap the stick in a bit of a cotton ball to soften it. Apply cuticle cream to the cuticle area to soften and moisturize the cuticles. Use the pumice stone on the sole and back of the heel to remove any rough skin. Rinse your foot and generously apply moisturizer.

Repeat on the other foot.

If you do not wish to paint your toenails, you can stop here or after step 4.

STEP 4 (OPTIONAL)

If you have the time and inclination, soothe your feet with self-massage. Grasp and squeeze the foot. Rub up and down the ankle, and press your fingers from the top of the foot into the knuckles of the toes. Your longest nerve, the sciatic, harbors negativity and stress. The saddle of the foot is its base, so make circles with your thumb on one side and four fingers on the other side. You'll be amazed how good this one area of your body will feel.

STEP 5

Twist the facial tissue so it's a rope. Weave it between your toes to separate them. You can also use toe separators, which are sold in most beauty supply stores. If the nail polish seems hard, it's okay to run it under very hot water to thin it. Dip the brush against the side of the bottle so the polish won't drip or be too thick. Starting at the cuticle, put a stripe of the polish down the center and then on each side of the nail. Remove mistakes quickly with a tissue over your fingernail. Two coats of polish and one top coat are classic. A blow dryer can be used to speed up the drying.

For winter holidays, gold-colored nail polish is great. For fall, try something muted. Pinks are great for spring. Nobody will notice how nice your toes look if you only wear the same shade month after month. Once in a while experiment with Granny Smith apple, aquamarine, lavender, or the latest new color. I like the O-P-I brand of polish because it lasts. You may have a knack for pedicures or you may not, but your toes will look bright and neat if you are careful. My advice is to leave the French manicure to the experts!

Let us not mock a man who kisses our feminine foot. The generators of these tired jokes about foot fetishists were attempting to shroud the beauty and sex appeal of this appendage. I think many women, when they see how flexible their babies' feet are, and how tender and kissable, get over the inhibition about caressing a foot. I love the idea that my guy's feet are heavily callused from running marathons, and where my feet are slender and flat, his are broader and have this sexy high arch.

A footbath is a treat for his feet too. If they are soft and smell of something herbal, as well as pliable from being relaxed, you have no excuse not to love him from head to toe.

It seems to me that the reason we go to the effort to have a pretty pair of feet is to uncover them. Your feet canoodle his feet and you discover his arch, the curve from his toes up to the top of the foot, or his ankles, or just the energy throbbing in his feet when you hold them.

Finally, as I looked at feet, I thought of Taoism, the world's religion we most identify with walking a path. I consulted with William Wei, senior instructor of the Universal Tao, who splits his time between the West Coast and northern Thailand, and has taught Taoism in more than thirty countries, for his understanding of feet and their particular energy.

Wei points out that feet wearing shoes contact the earth without any give and take, but bare feet touch a surface and yield to it. The yielding strengthens them and sets up a better energy flow with the whole body, so we should leave our feet bare as much as possible to cultivate good health. Reflexology is derived from ancient methods of foot massage: Reflex zones crisscross the body, with certain body parts and organs linked to areas of the feet and hands. Pressure is used to promote energy flow and alleviate symptoms caused by blockage of the energy paths. You don't have to understand this complex system to apply its methods. Wei says massaging especially sensitive points on a man's foot coddles him and brings him joy. Try an inch forward from the heel on the inside of the foot. Often reflexology "maps" are the same (mirrored) for both feet, and sometimes a connection is where you expect it—like the shoulder point being at the "shoulder" of the foot outside the little toe, or the waist being at the halfway point. An awareness of the most sensitive points of our feet is valuable knowledge whether you are massaging your feet against the rim of the tub or in the sand at the beach, or caressing your lover. For detailed guidance on how your hands and feet "speak" to different areas of the body and how to practice reflexology to benefit you or your loved ones, check out Kevin and Barbara Kunz's *Hand and Foot Reflexology: The Unique Self-Health Approach to Wellness* (HarperCollins, 1986).

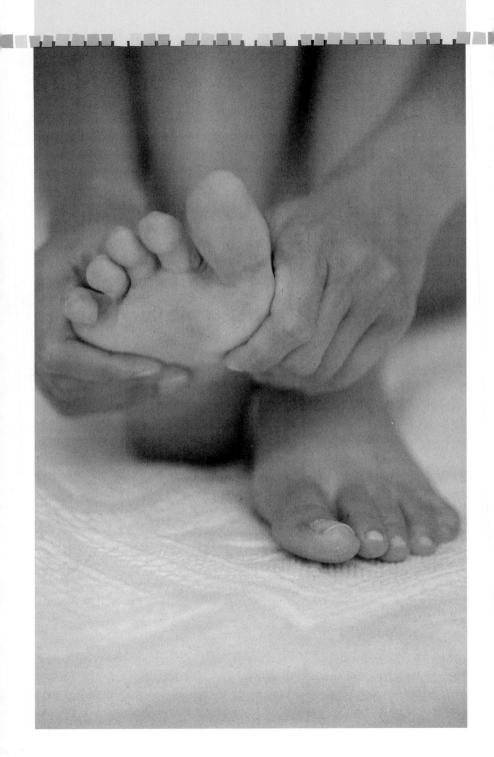

Foot Massage

YOUR KNEES MAY hurt because your feet are the problem. Your calves may be tight because of your shoes. If your knees hurt, your hips hurt, and your whole body is thrown off. Nothing makes tired feet feel better than a good massage.

Too busy for massage therapy? You don't have to have a diploma to take ten minutes for massage with your partner in the evening. These three invaluable massage techniques are really easy. The person receiving the massage lies prone. 1. Pull slowly and firmly on the ankles of both feet at the same time, raising the legs slightly. 2. Grasp and squeeze the feet over the ankles. 3. Press your thumb into the sole a little toward the toes from the arch. Repeat on the other foot.

Here is a simple pressure point trick that hails from reflexology. There is a lot of benefit in the simple idea of applying pressure, holding, releasing, and then repeating the pressure.

Start with these three moves; for each use your thumb and forefinger as a vise. Grasp the back of one ankle at a time and hold for five to eight seconds. Press with your thumb, giving the movement full concentration. Breathe, close your eyes once you latch on, and indent further until you feel your circulatory system pipe up, "Hey, what's doing?" Release your hold and repeat with the other ankle. Now grasp and hold the saddle of the foot, just past the ankle. This is the extremity of the biggest nerve in your body, the sciatic nerve. Hold tightly for 5 to 8 seconds and release. Now press in the fleshy part between your big toe and second toe, keeping your thumb flat. Hold for 5 seconds. Repeat on the opposite foot.

Your next trick is to move upside down with your feet. Lie with your head on a pillow, and elevate your feet against a wall as high as they will go. The backs of your legs should touch the wall, and your buttocks should nestle into the base of the wall. This is not a workout exercise, ladies, so stop flailing and just relax. You're going to do it every night because it has such a beneficial effect.

Part of why you love the beach is walking on the sand and curling your toes into its gritty smoothness. If a day at the beach is merely a thought on the horizon, pile up three pillows and prance on them. Your heels and arches will regale. This easy fatigue buster is best done with the most insubstantial pillows. After doing this you will never again wonder why children scatter pillows and dance around on them; it makes their growing feet feel so good.

Self-feathering is truly a trick. If you are diligent about doing it regularly, it may reduce cellulite and keep new cellulite from occurring. Sit down on your bed. Apply a runny lotion to your feet and legs all the way up. I like to mix one-third baby oil with two-thirds Williams-Sonoma Hand Lotion with Essence of Lavender. Starting with either leg, work slowly up the leg from toes to upper thigh. Draw your fingers up at either side and grasp lightly, then "feather" up using a movement like a harpist's so your fingers spread, catch the flesh, and then bounce off it. Then repeat on the opposite leg. This relaxes muscles, removes toxins, and increases circulation.

I love to give massages or receive them. But I feel like a one-armed paperhanger if I try to give a massage to myself. It seems like singing myself a lullaby to get to sleep! I make an exception only for these massages. Here is a foot massage (done lying down) that's just play but very soothing. Anchor the heel of your left foot on the top of your right foot, between the big toe and the fourth toe. Flex up and down the left foot that is supported. Once you are feeling easy about the position, rise off the left foot and work your right foot's toes around the sides and back of your left ankle. Then return the left foot to the cradle of the right foot and hold. Switch feet and repeat.

STONE MASSAGE

The perfect self-massage is stone massage. Using ancient stones on your body can be very evocative. Either order massage stones of black basalt, which retain heat and are oily smooth, or collect your own smooth, heavy-ish stones. You need three stones about three inches long and four stones the size of quarters.

Put the stones into a pot of boiling water, then turn off the heat and prepare your legs and feet with massage cream. After ten minutes, scoop the stones out of the hot water with a big slotted spoon and dry them with a towel. If you use basalt stones, they will keep the heat. You may want to use one big stone first, and go back later for the other six.

Lubricate the biggest stone with my basic no-stick mixture of two-thirds lotion and one-third baby oil. Squeeze a washcloth with hot water over your legs and let the water run all over your legs, letting the water cover your legs and feet. First test the stone against your knee to make sure it's not too hot. Rub the stone slowly up and down your calves, your inner thighs, and the tops of your feet. Then rest your feet on a raised pile of pillows or stack of books covered with a towel. Put one stone under each arch and the little stones on the fleshy parts of the bottoms of your feet just below the toes.

You can have your feet massaged to better health by a certified massage therapist. The therapist will look at your ligaments, nerves, and tendons, and get you to the point where you are pain free.

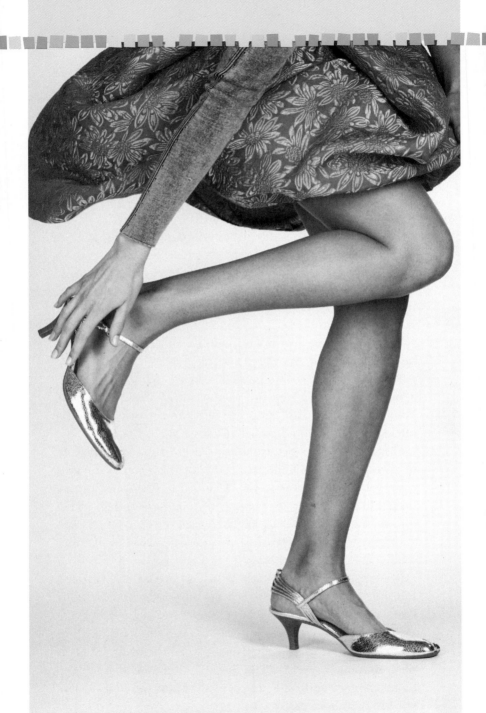

Shoes

A SHORT HISTORY OF THE SHOE

As extensions of our legs, shoes—particularly high heels—evoke sex appeal. Unfortunately, women as well as men have sacrificed comfort for fashion throughout the ages. In the 1500s Italian women wore *chopines*—shoes with thick pedestals of cork or wood—sometimes as high as eighteen inches. Marie Antoinette was executed in high heels, and Louis XIV wore five-inch heels decorated with miniature battle scenes.

The high heel developed in the sixteenth century from the wedged shoe and *chopine*. By the seventeenth century heels were a predominant feature in both men's and women's shoes. During the eighteenth century men's shoes became flat and were made of plain black leather, while women's shoes had intricate embroidery, bands of metallic braid, ribbon, and buckle ties.

Boots with elastic sides, buttons, or laces were fashionable in the nineteenth century for both men and women. Women's shoes had low heels and were made of silk, leather, or satin, with ribbon ties. Two-inch heels returned in the late nineteenth century, and some shoe styles were named after actresses, such as the Langtry, for the actress Lillie Langtry.

The First World War brought more functional footwear as women replaced men in factories and other workplaces.

Shoe manufacturers stressed dependable quality or comfort rather than style or glamour.

During World War II shoe designs were spartan. Open-toed shoes were banned as unsafe, and heels could be no more than one inch high. Most shoes were made of inferior-grade leather, cork, wood, or rubber. More feminine shoe designs emerged after the war and continued to thrive, with peep toes and higher heels. Marilyn Monroe personified sex appeal in *The Seven Year Itch* wearing high-heeled sling-back sandals with her pleated white halter dress. However, by the late 1950s, lower heels and long-toed shoes were fashionable.

The 1960s woke up the fashion world, and footwear became more daring than ever. Mod, space-age shoes and boots were made of plastic and other synthetic fabrics. Who can forget Jane Fonda in the 1968 film *Barbarella,* wearing thigh-high black-and-white patent-leather boots?

Platforms and wedge heels came back yet again in the 1970s, with soles made of cork, rope, plastic, or wood. Shoe styles tamed in the 1980s and '90s, with more delicate stiletto heels and pointed toes, like those by Manolo Blahnik, to complement the padded-shoulder power look. Extreme shoe fashions returned briefly in the 1990s, when the shoe designer Patrick Cox created six-inch platforms, but Vivienne Westwood topped these with her twelve-inch blue "mock-croc" platforms, which made the supermodel Naomi Campbell fall on a Paris runway.

Today's shoes are a blend of the past—platforms, wedges, stilettos, and flats. Even sports shoes are sexy, with bright colors and streamlined styles. Although shoe designs may change, the sexiness of the high heel is timeless.

SHOE ADVICE

The scene has changed, but shoe high fashion is just as crazy. We look for the most cushioned sneakers and then wear pointed-toe shoes that distort the shape of our feet.

Your feet look better when you are comfortable. You cannot look good in jeans or pants in the same shoes that you wear with a dress. Jeans and pants go with shoes that "say" practical, not dainty and dressy. Don't worry about wearing shoes that are too exciting or too young. Fashionable women would buy some of the adorable shoes from the children's department if they could!

Living as a child a town away from the Château de Versailles, I used to feel sorry for the noblemen forced by the king's fashions to wear heeled shoes that trailed masses of colored ribbons. Now I see it differently: Maybe dressing in ostentation was a fun revolt against autocracy. My daughter Emma, who just passed the New York State Bar, says that, in the corporations in D.C. where she has worked, "Exciting shoes are a safe way to make an outrageous fashion statement. In the corporate culture you are very limited in what you can wear, but it's still acceptable to veer off as an individual with your footwear. An attorney who's limited to dark suits at client meetings can express herself with Pradas shaded from hot pink to red. Flashy footwear is noticed and liked, considered okay if from the desk up you look like a corporate lawyer."

Here are a few principles of shoe buying I recommend. Shop for shoes in the afternoon, when your feet have swelled a bit, sometimes a significant amount. Buy shoes in which you can wiggle your toes. Ask the shoe seller to bring out a size bigger, even if you think the size you have on is okay. Powder your feet when you are going bare legged for a whole day or long evening, because your feet should glide inside the shoes, not stick.

Last, even if your fashion shoes fit, free your feet for a

couple hours each day. You can do this by padding around barefoot or by wearing exercise sandals, such as Birkenstocks. These can actually give your feet happiness while you go about your normal routine.

A few easy tricks are all you need to ease foot fatigue. If you build them into your life rather than stick them in that emergency ward/crisis part of your brain, they will enhance your whole being. Keep up the oxygen level in the appendages that suffer the most punishment in our daily lives. If you wait until they're overtired or the blood is pooling in your feet, or your ankles swell (even the merest amount), it's too late to restore them. Perform these tricks regularly; they are so easy.

Here are more tips that I recommend for preventing and easing foot pain and fatigue:

- Flex your toes when you wait in a line.

- For part of the day wear shoes that massage your feet. (Dr. Scholl's or the Australian brand called Maseur are good choices.)

- Slippers should be roomier than your day shoes and be made with high-quality materials and a very soft lining.

- Don't run on concrete.

- Keep one comfy pair of old match-anything shoes in the trunk of your car and another in a drawer at the office to change into if your shoes are hurting.

- Wear open-toed shoes when you can, and wiggle your toes.

- Be conscious of your feet so you can realize before misery sets in that they hurt. Look for opportunities to kick your shoes off or to sit down.

- Check out benches in museums and chairs at big parties because nothing will hurt your feet the way standing at attention does.

- If your feet are freezing, warm them up, and if they feel overheated stick them in a basin with a few ice cubes and some bath oil. Foot fatigue can result from extreme temperatures.

- Include a light massage when you moisturize your feet in the morning or the evening.

BOOT BUYING GUIDE

You see boots that will be great walking through a snowy woods or clicking across Central Park South. You are wearing shorts or office clothes. The most important thing when buying boots is your practical imagination of when you are actually going to wear them. Imagine them with pants, your peacoat, or dressy clothes. Ever bought boots that sit unworn for so long you worry about flushing out the cobwebs and scorpions when you haul them out . . . to move them to a different closet? Vow to wear them—if possible, right away.

Here are my hints for a successful boot-buying experience:

- Slim boots are elegant. Bright rubber boots are amusing. Arctic-looking boots are fun. Just don't get blah boots!

- Take a pair of athletic socks when you shop for boots. Your feet need the breathing space they give.

- Flex the soles of the boots you're considering. Even rugged boots should have soles that flex.

- Think about waterproofing: Do you need it? Probably. If the instructions on the boots suggest a boot-protecting silicone, buy and use it preseason.

- If you insist on pointy-toe boots, be sure your toes don't smash into the tips.

- No matter what the style of boots, they should have no-slip soles.

- Ask the salesperson to bring you one size higher than you think you wear and try those boots on first. If you swim in them, go down a size. If they feel roomy, they are the right size; snug boots cannot accommodate the normal swelling of feet in the course of a day.

- The top of the boot should not cut your leg. Check the stitching, fit, and lining at the top. If there is a zipper, is it well-protected so it will not abrade your skin?

- Check that the boot doesn't choke your ankle.

- The insulation should be of similar warmth all the way up. Poor design is sometimes reflected in very warm boot tops and thin leather around the feet.

- When you walk, your foot should be encased in the boot and not rub at the ankle.

Look down at the shoes we mostly wear into the world. They are sensible—the Adidas and the Birkenstocks. But when we want to be sexy, nothing does it better than a heel. Put on shoes with high heels, and you lift your calves, your back arches, your chest becomes prominent. Your whole posture says nothing less that "I am a woman." In a way that straight guys simply don't get, questions of heels or flats and ties or buckles affect a woman's persona. And isn't the ultimate reason we love the shoes that are good for us that they keep our feet healthy to wear the sexy ones?

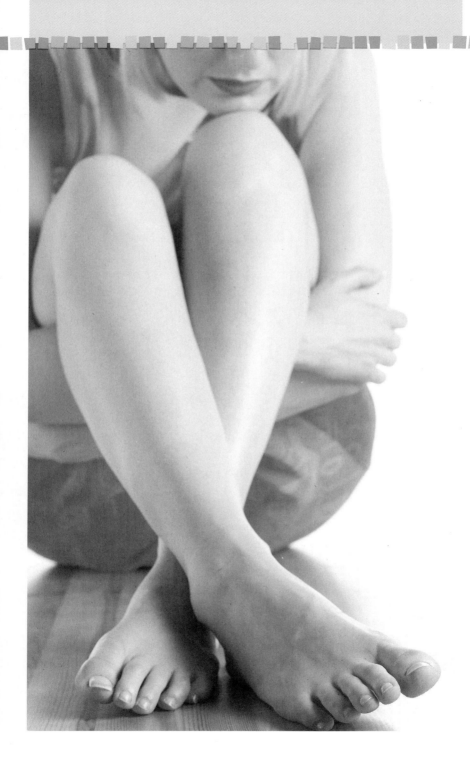

$\mathcal{F}oot$ $\mathcal{C}are$ $\mathcal{A}dvice$

CALLUSES AND BUNIONS

Women often develop calluses at the tips of their toes. Callus tissue builds up as a result of hammertoes, toes curled under. There are simple ways of dealing with a callus problem. First, you can use a softer insole in the forward area of any shoe where your toes rub. Moisturizing creams or lotions can hydrate the skin *and* decrease friction. There are callus creams or lotions with safe-to-use skin-diluting acids that hydrate more powerfully. These products, over-the-counter derivatives of urea or lactic acid, help slough away calluses and encourage the skin to turn over more quickly so calluses don't build up.

A more complicated way of dealing with calluses on the tips of your toes is an orthotic device that balances the tendons and muscles in your feet. These "intrinsic" muscles are mainly responsible for keeping the toes straight, and in a normal foot they fine-tune movement. When these muscles tire, as they do in adulthood, they allow those long muscles of your leg that extend and flex the toes to take over, and hammertoe deformities can result.

If you are prone to foot trouble: Before shoes become rigid, put orthotics (prescription foot supports) in shoes that allow space to place them. They should have metatarsal pads or even toe crests—little lifts that go under your toes to relax the contraction.

How we walk in our shoes and the interface of the shoe and foot can also cause knobs to develop on the tops of the toes, referred to as hammertoes. They may become red and swollen because the tissue beneath the skin is inflamed. A callus then forms on top of the center of the toe. If this is happening to you, it's time to change your shoes! Increasing the height of the toe box of your shoes, or wearing shoes slightly longer than normal (without sacrificing comfort or fit) helps. If the bunion on the big toe becomes more rigid, it may require surgery.

Bunions can bulge on the knuckle of the big toe. Bunionettes can develop behind the small toe. The first treatment option is to find shoes that better accommodate the width of your feet. Wider shoes will prevent the redness and irritation, and eliminate small metatarsal and big metatarsal bump irritation. Orthotics help keep the metatarsals from splaying or spreading apart. If you try these just for running and other aerobic sports, you should see improvement. Some people are prone to bunions because of heredity.

For more critical conditions, surgical procedures have become incredibly refined and effective. Says Conneticut podiatrist and foot surgeon Dr. Andrew H. Rice, "Often women return to the shoes they liked to wear and to all the activities they did prior to the bunions. Bunionettes respond to the same types of procedures, where we realign the bones or remove a section of bone." Just make sure the surgeon you choose is board-certified in the field.

TOENAILS

According to Dr. Rice, "Toenails are a sign of beauty in many cultures, and are enameled and decorated. When the nails become abnormally thick or discolored, people feel unhealthy, whereas in reality nails change only because of the trauma of being in shoes all our lives." He gives several ways to improve the looks of our nails. When the nails become thickened, or appear to have debris beneath them, several treatments are available. Topically, Penlac brush-on laquer can soften the nail and get rid of fungus. It has to be used for an extended time, and the nail has to be pared of any thickened portions, but Penlac has no side effects. Success rates vary and may be lower than those of some oral medications. Lamisil and Sporanox are oral medications that will cure more that 50 percent of the people treated. These are quite safe, but your blood count and liver function have to be monitored by a doctor while you are taking them. There are also medications to soften nails and help them lose ugly thickness. Softening agents like fungoid tincture, Keralac, and Carmol work on the keratin tissue of the nails.

The predisposition to develop nail fungus is increased by polishing the nails. Nails absorb water; they are porous. When we bathe, shower, or swim, our skin gets wrinkly but also softer. When we have enamel on our nails, the water that soaks them has no place to evaporate. Dr. Rice recommends that you remove nail polish frequently and let your nails breathe. He says, "If you are going to wear work or dress shoes for the next five days of your workweek and your toenails are not going to be exposed to the air, take your nail polish off. Let your nails breathe better."

The area between your toes is a common place to harbor fungus. You can decrease it by using over-the-counter topical medications such as Lotrimin. There are prescription medicines like Loprox, Spectazole, Naftin, and many others that will eliminate fungal infections as well. If you have ever had this problem, be sure to dry your toes well after bathing. If you use a public shower at the gym, also be sure to wear shower shoes.

PAIN

Several causes of heel pain are contraction of the Achilles tendon, which tightens an arch structure called the plantar fascia, injury, arthritis, and improper conditioning. Heel pain often occurs when you go barefoot for a prolonged period after wearing mostly high heels. For example, you'll probably have some discomfort wearing flip-flops all day on a beach vacation if you usually wear high or even mid heels.

Ever had a stabbing pain in your arch? Dr. Rice says these can be virtually prevented by limiting how many hours you walk in sheerly glamorous shoes, and by engaging in an exercise regimen for legs and feet that is coupled with stretching exercises. He says, "Today many women don't take the time at the end of a workout to stretch. If they integrate yoga or Pilates exercises after they do aerobics or weight training, their feet will benefit enormously."

DR. RICE'S FOOT EXERCISES

Dr. Rice's whole series of foot exercises takes about ten minutes. If you do the series several times a week, he promises you'll have more alert, flexible, and shapely, and less accident-prone feet throughout your life. If you think your feet are asking for too much, do these nine exercises once and then consider which will fit in with your daily activities.

1. ANKLE-FOOT-HEEL AND PLANTAR FASCIA STRETCH
Standing with the ball of one foot on a stair, reach for the lower step with your heel until you feel a stretch through the arch. Hold several seconds. Relax. Repeat 12 times. Then repeat with the other foot.

2. PLANTAR FASCIA STRETCH
Sitting in a chair, grab your ankle and pull your foot toward your buttocks. Pick your heel up so you feel a stretch in your arch. Hold 10 seconds. Repeat 10 times. Then repeat with the other foot.

3. HEEL-CORD WALL STRETCHES
Place your hands on a wall in front of you, supporting your weight on one leg. Extend the other leg behind your body with your heel flat on the floor and lean forward.

Hold for 5 seconds. Repeat 10 times on each leg. It is best if you do this twice a day.

4. TOE FLEXION-EXTENSION STRETCHES
While sitting, gently grasp the toes of one foot and curl them under, then straighten them. Hold while straight for 10 seconds. Repeat 2 times per set. Then repeat with the other foot. This exercise will alleviate and prevent hammertoes and cramping foot muscles.

5. FOOT CIRCLES
Sit in a chair with your feet flat on the floor two to three feet in front of you. Lift the fronts of your feet high up, so only your heels remain on the floor. Slowly rotate the front parts of your feet clockwise, making complete circles.

Repeat several times, then rotate in the opposite direction.

6. FOOT CURL Sit in a chair with your feet flat on the floor. Point your toes inward and lift your arches, with the outer edges of your feet remaining on the floor. Then curl your toes under. Hold 3 seconds, then straighten again. Repeat several times.

7. TOE ABDUCTION Lie on your back with your feet flat and together and your toes pointing up. "Unhinge" your feet and as you do spread your toes wide and hold. Repeat several times.

8. TOE FLEXION Sit in a chair with your feet flat on the floor. Place a thick book under the bottoms of your feet. Slide your feet forward so your toes extend over the front edge of the book. Slowly bend your toes downward, then raise them. Repeat a few times.

9. TOE EXTENSION Sit in a chair with your feet flat on the floor. Slowly lift your toes, keeping the bottoms of your feet on the floor. Lower your toes to the floor and repeat a few times. (This makes toe joints more supple.)

The upside of these exercises is that they will add grace and flexibility to your feet and help you perform better in all sports. The downside is that since we aren't used to doing foot exercises, it's an unpleasant comeuppance to realize how stiff, needy, and overcivilized our feet have become. Be a cheerleader for your feet and tell them the only way is up.

If, on the other foot, you think your gams are asking for too much attention and time, do these exercises as I do. As you go through the complete series several times in order, figure out how they will fit into your daily activities. Then do the exercises regularly but piecemeal, i.e., several when you sit at lunch, others in the gym, and soon. If you explain to a guy that he will have fewer injuries and perform better at his favorite sports by sprucing up his feet, you may gain the motivation of doing them duo. Or take the exercises, a beach chair, and a towel to the seaside (as I did) to imprint them in your body and mind.

Conclusion

HAVE YOU EVER wondered why walking on a sandy beach makes you feel all-over heavenly, or why when you visit a new city and walk your legs off, it electrifies you body and soul despite the fatigue? When worked hard, the powerful muscles of our legs correspondingly invigorate our hearts, lungs, and nervous systems. When, through a spa-type treatment, minerals, salts, and moisturizing elements are absorbed through the skin into the legs and feet, superficial blood vessels throughout the body dilate, and stress hormones like cortisol decrease, causing relaxation in every cell. When we emphasize stretching and do aerobic exercise, not only do we strengthen our legs and make them more supple on every level but we rejuvenate our whole bodies.

Thank your legs for requiring so little to be gorgeous and stay young! Through a well-rounded exercise program of aerobics, weight lifting, and yoga (or comparable activities); a diet that includes nutrients for circulation and the skin; sunscreen when in intense exposure; massage or self-massage; and home or professional spa treatments including soaking, exfoliation, and moisturizing, we beautify our legs and feet. The routine is what counts; through it we can have more toned, smooth, shapely, and strong legs year after year. It's nice if you are also self-analytic enough to see when an enhancement—from a buttery mask, overnight foot socks or callus sloughing to laser touch-ups for little, resistant flaws—is called for.

Now that you've read this book, here's a plan that you can use for a lifetime—without going crazy!

IF YOU'RE UNDER THIRTY-FIVE:

- Select a hair removal method that works for you.
- Use sunscreen when you are in the sun for prolonged periods.
- Take care of any fungal problem and use tea tree oil or an antifungal spray if you share a bed or bathroom with anybody.
- Firm your calves with pinpoint exercises.
- Elongate your entire legs with dance, yoga, or Pilates.
- Do an aerobic exercise like running for your thighs.
- Once a week, give yourself a home spa treatment.
- Use a moisture mask when your skin shows signs of drying.
- Indulge in regular pedicures.

AFTER YOUR CHILDBEARING YEARS:

- If spider or varicose veins do not go away, by using vitamin K or Dr. Perricone's cream, and you still have them within several years after having babies, investigate laser treatment with a dermatologist or vascular surgeon.
- Exercise to tone your thighs and buttocks.
- Have regular pedicures.
- Use body butter on dry trouble spots.
- Take antioxidants to repair collagen and elastin.
- Increase the elasticity of your skin with bath salts.
- If age spots develop, see a dermatologist for laser magic.

AND TWO MORE THINGS AT ANY AGE

- Love your legs for everything they can do.
- And take a big hint from the German-born film star Marlene Dietrich, who said, "The average man is more interested in a woman who is interested in him than he is in a woman—any woman—with beautiful legs."

Shopping Guide

THERE ARE MANY wonderful and many to-be-avoided leg and foot beauty products on the market. Bargain shopping can result in a discouraging array of sticky, perfumy, ineffectual gels, creams, and so forth. Here are my recommendations:

LINES OF HIGH, CONSISTENT QUALITY AND MODERATE PRICE

- Caswell-Massey
- Erbaviva
- Get Fresh
- Kneipp
- Tipton Charles

SHOWER GELS

I choose shower gel by scent and on sale, but if you are committed to showers and like to experiment, there are a few interesting twists on shower products, such as these:

- Bliss's Super-Eucalyptus Smoother (preshower body softening mask)
- Bliss's Lemon Peel Body Polishing Scrub Cream
- Aromafloria's Stress Less Phytobath Gel

SEA SALTS AND SOAKS

- Erbaviva products are truly pure and gentle, and free from artificial fragrances, additives, dyes, and animal testing. All their high-quality oils are in a carrier oil (base) of organic almond, safflower, and jojoba oils. I highly recommend their moisturizing bath salts: Embrace (citrus, cedar, and jasmine, designed to gently decrease cellulite on legs); Awaken (to revive, with melissa, lemongrass, and rose); Relax (calming, blending lavender, rose, and neroli), and Breathe (www.erbaviva.com; phone 877-372-2848).
- Aromafloria Muscle Soak (eucalyptus, peppermint, and lemongrass)

- Tipton Charles salts in Pomegranate, Apricot-Basil, Acqua Blue, and Creamsicle (phone 800-340-1075, 718-433-3866; fax 718-433-4640)
- Hot salt scrub (self-heating) by Bliss
- Molton Brown Sea Moss Stress-Relieving Hydrosoak
- Davies Gate Lavender Oatmeal and Rice Bath Salts (www.daviesgate.com)
- Davies Gate Powder Sugar Bath Soak (in Peppermint, Cinnamon, and Sweet Orange)
- Green Valley Aromatherapy Ltd. (www.57aromas.com, phone 877-572-7662)

SCRUBS (EXFOLIATING)
- Douglas Beauty System Salt and Sugar Body Scrub
- Sweet orange and spearmint sugar scrub by Bliss

BATH OILS AND MORE
- Tipton Charles bubble bath in Pomegranate, Acqua Blue, and Creamsicle
- Tipton Charles bath oil
- Tipton Charles shea butter pads to toss into the bath
- Aromafloria Bath Fizz in pomegranate and lemongrass
- Davies Gate Lemon-Thyme Nutrient-Rich Foaming Bath
- Do Not Disturb Lavender Bath Gel (www.dodisturb.com)
- Douglas Beauty System Silky Bath Oil with ylang-ylang

MOISTURIZERS TO SMOOTHE AND SOFTEN LEGS
- Erbaviva Body Lotion. Similar blends as their moisturizing bath salts
- Molton Brown Inspiring Wild-Indigo Body Lotion
- Caswell-Massey Body Lotion in almond-honey and other scents
- Kiehl's Deluxe Hand and Body Lotion
- Yardley Silky Sail's Body Cream with sea kelp

Rich and thickly textured—you can often guess these by the fact that they come in tubs not tubes:
- Kiehl's Crème de Corps Riches
- Mor's Grapefruit Body Balm
- Do Not Disturb Lavender Spa Cream
- Douglas Relaxing Body Cream with ylang-ylang

SPRAY-ON TAN
- Sally Hansen Airbrush Legs (drugstores)
- Trish McEvoy—Legs only spray tan (212-988-7816)
- Air Stocking (www.airstocking.com/usa)
- Bloom's Aloha Body Shimmer Cream (Sephora)

SHAVING AND HAIR REMOVAL
- Gillette for Women Venus Divine razor. An enhanced version of the popular Venus razor with aloe moisture strips and an easy-glide oval cartridge.
- Kiehl's Close-Shaverettes "Simply Mahvelous Legs" Shave Cream
- Kiehl's After-Shave Lotion
- Sally Hansen's Spa Gel Hair Remover
- Tipton Charles Shave Lotion (instead of foam, a gentle lotion with extracts of thyme, chestnut, cucumber, and rosemary)

LEG MAKEUP
- Jergens Shimmer
- Air Stocking's Jewel
- Clarins Spray Huile Irisée Après Soleil

VITAMINS AND NUTRIENTS
- Nu Visage's Complete Leg and Vein Therapy Regimen with oral supplement to strengthen skin and veins, and leg cream; made with OPC (866-688-4724)
- E•lix•r's tonic for circulation is taken in a tasty tablespoon each day. (www.elixirtonics.com)
- Vitamin B complex, vitamins E and K, coenzyme Q_{10}

GOING DEEPER: TONING, CELLULITE, AND SPIDER VEINS
- CoQ_{10} to prevent aging of skin (often taken daily in two or three small doses)
- Vitamins B_2, B_3, and B_{12} for skin
- Folic acid for vessels and to prevent leg cramps
- Vitamin C for collagen
- Vitamin E for skin
- Vitamin K for circulation

- Shiseido Body Creator aromatic toning gel
- Body Toning by Dr. N. V. Perricone
- Aromafloria Healing Waters Tighten and Tone Treatment Gel
- Hyrogel Aromatique (decongests) by Darphin
- Clarins Extra-Firming Body Care (moisturizing and firming, with peach, water lily, and Amazonian bocoa)
- Clarins Body Lift Advanced Cellulite Control
- Dr. Perricone's Anti-Spider Vein, Legs
- DDF Refining Body Treatment (caffeine, ginseng, and ginkgo for lymphatic drainage and to boost blood flow), High Thighs Cellulite Fighting Serum, and High Thighs Slimmer Scrub from Bliss (888-243-8825)
- Streiveichten
- Mei camellia seed oil (www.victani.com)
- Algotherm's Firming and Slimming Gel
- Erbaviva's Stretch Mark Oil and Stretch Mark Cream, combining shea butter, sea buckthorn, and feverfew extracts with oils of carrot, rose, and avocado. Designed especially for mothers to be, this product is great for those going through periods of weight gain and has even been known to reduce wrinkles and treat dry skin! Erbaviva recommends you apply the cream in the morning and the oil at night.

FOOT CREAM
- Emu Neat Feet (a cream with aloe vera, tea tree oil, and emu oil). Available from Massage Warehouse.
- Carmol

MASSAGE CREAM
- Santa Barbara Massage Cream (in clary sage–lavender, eucalyptus, lavender, and ylang-ylang-orange). Available from Massage Warehouse.

KITS
- Glow and Go Kit (Spa Scrub/Dry Body Oil Spray/Tighten and Tone Treatment Gel) by Aromafloria (www.aromafloria.com)